C000004115

THE WOMAN

Who Wouldn't Die

by

Don Lucey

UCT™ Publications

Published by
UCT™ Publications
Suite 125
116 Commercial Road
Swindon
Wiltshire SN1 5BD, UK
www.thewomanwhowouldntdie.com
email: DonLucey1180@aol.com

A CIP catalogue record for this book
is available from the British Library

ISBN 0-9541100-0-5

UCT™ Publications

CONTENTS

ACKNOWLEDGEMENTS

I would like, above all, to thank Rebecca, my daughter, for her love, understanding and support without which I would not have been able to research, write and publish this book.

My thanks also go to the nursing colleague, a friend of Christine's, who alerted us to the misreported 'positive' smear in her hospital records. Without this information Chris would have had even less chance to fight for her survival and an even shorter life expectancy. No compensation claim would have been possible.

I am also indebted to our two medical experts, Professor Roger Cotton and Pat Soutter MD, who helped us to build our case for compensation: and allowed me to present their medical reports to our lawyers. Specific thanks to Professor Cotton for his invaluable expertise in helping me to understand the development of cervical cancer and the rationale of the smear-testing programme.

Huge thanks go to the rehabilitation nurse, Verne Anne Convey, and to the nursing staff and others, who cared for and supported Chris throughout her illness.

Words are not sufficient to recognise the dedication and devotion of my dear friend, John Czul, our solicitor. He devoted many years of his life to the struggle to win justice for Christine. I am indebted to his wealth of legal knowledge and to his professional, calm, and meticulous approach, which finally resulted in victory against a faceless and bureaucratic system.

My grateful thanks to my first-draft editors, Doug Watts and Jenny Hewitt, who believed in my book, critiqued and revised my manuscript, and my editor, Judith Hampson, who restructured the text. Further thanks are due to Barbara Large, MBE FRSA, editorial consultant and to George Mann, George Mann Publications, for book layout and production. Thanks to all of you for your dedication, professionalism and for tirelessly working all hours to help me finish this task. Your words of encouragement and belief in the book lifted my spirits and kept me going at times when the task seemed impossible.

I extend my thanks to Marianne Crowley, Jane Warren, and everyone else who gave up their time, listened to me and helped me along the way. Your friendship has been and continues to be, invaluable.

Thanks to Helen Cooke, Director of Therapy at the Bristol Cancer Help Centre, for permission to print extracts from the Nutritional and Complementary Therapy programme.

Many professional colleagues and friends have helped bring this book to its completion, have combed through various drafts and have offered comments, criticism and advice. I have endeavoured to tell Chris's story as accurately as possible. Any errors that remain are, of course, entirely my own.

Don Lucey, September 2001

FOREWORD

When I first read the manuscript sent to me by Don Lucey I knew immediately this was a story that must be told. The production of this book not only pays respect to Christine Lucey for her bravery in fighting her illness for so long against horrendous odds, but also it represents a timely warning to all women of the need to be vigilant in monitoring their own health and not to give their power away to doctors by investing blind faith in them. Doctors are not infallible; they can and do make catastrophic mistakes.

Sometimes mistakes are understandable, even unavoidable. Not so in the tragic case of Christine Lucey. Christine need not have suffered what she suffered, probably not even a fraction of it. In all probability, she need not have died. A smear test taken as early as 1977 showed abnormal cells which were misreported by the hospital to Christine's GP. This smear test was not simply "clear" as reported to Christine and it should have been repeated: similarly, the smears taken in 1978 were reported as clear. Smears were not taken with the regularity they should have been, given the atypical cells that they showed. Two smear tests results were lost altogether and could not be subsequently reviewed by Professor Roger Cotton, Histopathologist, when he prepared evidence for the compensation claim.

I have read that evidence. It revealed that *ten years* after those first warning signs two smear tests, January and August, 1986, were taken which should have resulted in immediate referral to a gynaecologist. These were also reported as "clear" or "negative" to the patient. Professor Cotton subsequently examined these tests and determined that the cell changes in the smears at that time were serious but probably pre-invasive. Had Christine then been examined and referred for a biopsy, this would have revealed early cervical disease that could have been treated by laser, cryotherapy, diathermy or cone biopsy. The prognosis would then have been very good. Statistics for the treatment of cervical disease of this nature at this stage show no local recurrence in more than 95% of cases. The five-year survival rate after treatment is almost 100% with a very good prognosis thereafter.

There were also other warning signs that all was not well. In 1982 Christine was treated for abdominal pain that was diagnosed by her gynaecologist as endometriosis. In 1984, vaginal bleeding was diagnosed as a miscarriage. In 1986, an ovarian cyst, caused by fertility treatment, had to be removed. In 1987, during her pregnancy, she required emergency treatment for abdominal pain and vaginal bleeding. The smear test results, containing vital information, should have been elicited during all of this treatment.

Worse was to come. During physical examination while Christine was pregnant, her gynaecologist noted irregularities in the cervix and the presence of nodules. She was haemorrhaging at this time. Christine then told him that she had been recalled because of "funny cells" in some of her smears. Shortly afterwards in January, 1988, Rebecca was delivered by emergency Caesarean section. The operative surgeon recommended a cone biopsy after noting that the cervix felt 'woody'. The gynaecologist should, by now, have suspected cancer or pre-malignant changes in the cervix but he overruled the need for biopsy. Christine felt "reassured" that he did not consider it necessary.

Christine had two more smear tests in 1988 that were 'positive' on review, but which were reported as showing only severe inflammatory changes. One was taken by her gynaecologist, the other was taken in June by her GP who requested an urgent repeat on the grounds that Christine now had severe post-coital bleeding, a symptom of invasive cervical cancer and that other smears had been abnormal. This smear was severely abnormal, showing malignant cells in clumps and a cone biopsy should then have been an immediate requirement. Cone biopsy may well have shown pre-invasive cancer treatable by local procedures. It might however, have shown invasive carcinoma in the early stages, probably stage 1. Had it done so, a radical hysterectomy possibly followed by radiotherapy would have been carried out and if stage 1b, a survival rate at five years of 85%-95% with a very good prognosis thereafter. Christine's gynaecologist examined Christine in August, 1988, at the insistence of her GP. He found no cause for concern.

The bleeding, almost continuous after the birth of Rebecca, finally resulted in Chris being admitted to hospital as an emergency in January, 1989. Only then was cancer diagnosed and immediate radio and chemotherapy commenced. The partial hysterectomy subsequently performed was inadequate due to local extension of disease. The operation was not straightforward, yet the surgeons did not call for the requisite expertise. The cervix, which was the seat of the tumour and the lymph glands, which can carry cancerous cells away from the site of origin to other parts of the body, were not removed. In fact, no signs of malignancy were found in the tissue that *was* removed on May 1, 1989 but when a radical pelvic clearance procedure was carried out on December 6, 1989 residual cancer cells were found on microscopic examination in tissue outside the rectum and in the posterior wall of the bladder.

If any good can come out of such a catalogue of incompetence and subsequent suffering it can only be that the telling of the story can warn other women; can prevent other similar experiences. Don Lucey has worked tirelessly for three years, piecing together medical information, re-living the horror of those six years, in order to issue just such a warning.

We have to rely on the expertise of doctors but ultimately; we are also each responsible for our own health. Cervical smear tests should be conducted in Britain, according to DHS guidelines, *at least* every five years. Make sure you have them. Most districts offer them every three years. If they don't, you can request them.

If you are refused, you have the option of having interim smears done privately. Talk to your doctor or practice nurse about the results, ask to see them. You have the right. Make sure that they *are* actually negative if they are reported to you as such. If they contain abnormal cells, make sure you have a repeat test. If you cannot talk to your GP in a full and frank way, a discussion between adults in which you have as much authority as the doctor, it's your body, then you do have the right to change your GP. You also have the right to request referral to a female GP and a female specialist for women's medical issues.

Finally, if you suspect anything worrying in relation to your health, ask what tests are available that can put your mind at rest. If a test is offered to you, do take it, even when doctors may disagree about its necessity. Most tests have negative results and will allay your concerns. But there is no merit whatever in not knowing. If there is disturbing news then medical action can be taken. The sooner it is taken, the more likely it is to be life-saving.

Judith Hampson BSc PhD
Editor

AUTHOR'S PREFACE

I had waited six years for this day to arrive. It was Tuesday, 24 March, 1998. I was on my way to London on the 0705 train from my home in Swindon, Wiltshire. My briefcase contained documents that, in a few hours, would be used to provide evidence before Lord Justice Judge Alliott, a High Court judge in the Royal Courts of Justice, presiding in Court Thirteen.

In March, 1995, three years earlier, the defendants, the Ministry of Defence, had admitted liability in a case of medical negligence and it had seemed that the settlement would be speedy. My wife was suffering horrendously. They were responsible. They had admitted it. Settling then, out of court, would have shown her courtesy and compassion. It would have enabled Christine to have a better quality of life in the time she had left to live. She needed so much help with the disability she now had. Her dream was to be able to live without financial worry and to convert our home to make it more suitable for her daily needs.

Sadly, that dream never came true. She died before the settlement was made. The defendants later dragged the case all the way to the doors of the High Court.

Christine died in the hospital where she had begun her training as a young nurse: her life totally destroyed by the blunders of the medical profession. She had suffered for over six years. Her illness had wrecked our happy marriage.

This is our story. I have tried to tell it as Christine would have wanted it told. I hope that it will be of value to others.

I have learned that it is possible to come to terms with the most terrible tragedy; to rebuild a meaningful life. A case such as this requires justice not only to be done, but also to be seen to be done. With the publication of this book, it has been.

Don Lucey

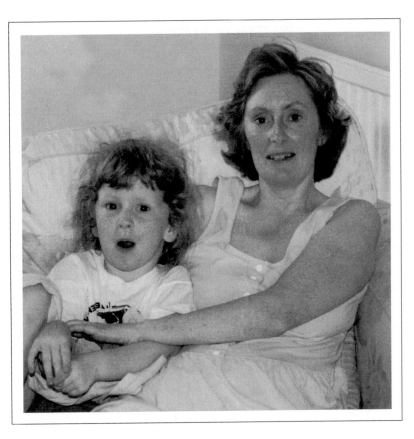

for Rebecca and Christine

ONE

*My wife, Christine, was bleeding to death
and there was nothing anyone could do to save her life*

In the end, Christine took fifteen hours to die. She bled to death – in hospital. Death should not happen this way; it should happen easily, painlessly. With dignity. In Christine's case, an uncomfortable and unsatisfactory death marked the end of a very long road of extreme and unnecessary suffering.

It is difficult to describe the feeling inside, when someone close to you has died. Those that have experienced a tragic loss know only too well that it changes one's life irrevocably. Everyone says that we move on, that time is a great healer. To a degree that depends on how close two people have been, how much they have shared. Chris and I had shared so very much more than most: the highs and the lows, the good memories and the bad. In particular, we had shared the trauma of six years of dealing with Christine's cancer. Together.

My first experience of death and bereavement was at the age of ten. I well remember the impact it made on me and my family when my father took his own life two days after Christmas in 1962. The abrupt end to my father's life and the tragic circumstances surrounding his death were to change my perception of contentment and happiness forever.

I was the one who found his body that freezing cold morning, while the rest of my family lay asleep. I was playing happily in the deep snow on the morning that I made my gruesome discovery. The landscape was free of footprints or tyre marks from Dad's tractor. Everything was clean and white and wonderful. I was the first to explore it all, stomping up and down in the fresh, crisp snow. I thought how my brothers and sisters would react when they charged out of the cottage a little later, complaining to each other, envious of me being the first to venture onto the virgin snow. There were no other sounds as I scrunched around on my own but I knew Mum would be awake because it was almost seven o'clock. She was always up at the same time every morning.

Before going indoors for breakfast, I threw a few snowballs at the barn door. I knew Dad was out here somewhere; he never stayed in bed in the mornings. My last snowball hit one of the large, rusting hinges and the door swung open.

I saw the lower part of his torso first. He was halfway up the wooden staircase that led to the hayloft. I expected him to shout at me, but he didn't move or say anything as the barn door opened. My curiosity tempted me to move closer: I wanted to find out what he was doing. I stepped into the barn and started to climb the stairs. He was bound to see me soon and then I'd probably get a good telling-off for being here, since we were only allowed to play in certain areas of the farm. The bales of straw and hay were stored in this barn and climbing on them was forbidden.

He was leaning against the wall, his left foot balanced precariously; the other dangled inches from the step below. His black hobnailed boots were covered in dust. He was wearing his usual work clothes: dark navy blue trousers and a black, heavy woollen jacket with string tied around the waist.

I didn't notice the rope around his neck as I moved towards him. It seemed he was sleeping, slouched against the wall like some drunken man. I squeezed past him, tiptoeing as quietly as I could for fear of waking him. He used to take his belt off sometimes and whip me and my brothers and sisters if we were naughty or argued with each other.

At that moment, my younger brother, James, ran in through the door, startling me. I turned and gestured him to be quiet, but he ran up the stairs towards me, pushing past me in the process.

Then we both panicked and ran past Dad's motionless form to the top. We were trapped. There was no way back. And besides, I didn't want to go back down the stairs. Dad was sure to leap on us and we would be punished.

Eventually though, I plucked up the courage and made my way back down the stairs, my brother following behind, holding tightly onto my coat. I still wanted to find out how deeply my father was asleep, so I kicked his foot to awaken him. His whole body twisted slowly towards me, the overhead beam creaking under his weight.

It was the noise that made me look up.

It took a split second for me to realise he was hanging. Quickly I turned to my brother but saw that he had already clambered back up the stairs and found a way out. He jumped from the open loft door to the ground below, his fall broken by bales of straw. I followed quickly behind, my legs kicking in mid-air as I dropped the twenty feet to land beside him.

My heart pounded as I ploughed my way through the deep snow, desperate to get to the cottage and tell my mother. She didn't believe me at first, She thought my story was a ploy to escape punishment for going into the barn. I should have known better and stayed outside.

She had to believe me! "Mum, Mum," I said, "he's in the barn. *He's got a rope around his neck!*"

I remember that we all stood outside the barn. Dad's body was still twisting slowly round and round. There was a lot of commotion after that.

My young, inquisitive mind had lured me to venture into the unknown that day, and the resultant emotional distress I endured, along with the shock of realising that my father had died by committing suicide, haunted me for months.

Fortunately, it did not have any long-term effect. My mother's love, devotion, and support, despite her own grief, gave me and my brothers and sisters the resilience to accept the tragedy. She would often encourage us to pray; her faith in God continued and she believed He would guide us through the remainder of our lives.

My father was forty-two years old when he died. He left no suicide note to explain the reasons for ending his own life. We left the farm only four weeks afterwards.

Our next home was ten miles away, a semi-detached council house in Avonmouth, a dockland area of Bristol choked with industrial pollution. For some reason I particularly remember the merchant seamen, mostly foreigners, who crowded the streets around the port, selling cheap bottles of alcohol and packets of Peter Stuyvesant cigarettes to wayward children.

Somehow we survived through those years. My mother never gave up. She kept her faith and determination. Her goal: simply to raise her eight children.

The search for adventure stayed with me for six years. I left school in 1968 and joined the British Army. I was sixteen years old.

*

I remember the first time that I met Christine on the evening of October 22. I was stationed in the Army Garrison of Tidworth. It was a Friday afternoon – the end of another week. The twelve-man dormitory near my room was the usual familiar sight: squaddies who were staying in camp collapsed on their beds, wondering how best to fill their spare time over the weekend.

Spirits were running high in Candahar Barracks, particularly in the dormitory. Several of us were getting ready to go out for the evening, when Taffy shouted in his West Glamorgan accent, "There's a party at the Medic's Club tonight. Who's coming, then?" He looked around, waiting for a response but everyone seemed to have suddenly found something very important to do.

"Well I'm going to the cash point to get some cash," he said finally, "does anyone want to come with me?" No one replied, except for an odd mumble here and there. He shrugged his shoulders and left the room to go on his own.

A few of us did go over to the Medic's Club, which was only a short distance from our barrack block. As usual, a frenzy of excitement buzzed about the place. It was the best unit club in the whole garrison. Everyone knew that Friday and Saturday nights were popular, most of the garrison's hospital staff were there. It was the only club that didn't have the usual boring group of predominantly male squaddies, who whinged all the time while consuming gallon upon gallon of lager.

This club was more respectable and friendlier. The downside was that everyone seemed to watch one another, which was often embarrassing, especially if an unfortunate friend failed in his attempt to woo a member of the opposite sex. Generally everyone would have a good laugh chatting up the nurses and the air was always thick with tales of rejections and successes, adding atmosphere to the place.

I was standing at the bar talking to a friend, a corporal, familiarly known as a full screw, in the Royal Army Medical Corps. Max Webster was a fellow Physical Training Instructor and something of an 'agony aunt' for the lads in the Royal Welsh Fusiliers. He had a penchant for smoking large cigars.

It was not long before Simon Elliott joined us. Single like me and totally outrageous, Simon was a young doctor with the rank of captain in the RAMC. He was an American, a loud-mouthed Yank, but he could get away with it. Everybody liked him. Simon was an accomplished entertainer, the typical life and soul of any party. With his arrival, the trio was complete: we were the best of friends.

The club was crowded; the three of us dominating the bar like the three bloody musketeers. In the background the music blared out Peter Frampton's *Baby I Love Your Way*. Suddenly, a group of girls appeared at the bar, laughing and obviously enjoying their evening.

Max and Simon were oblivious to them, but I became wedged in their midst. A northern accent caught my attention and as I turned towards a slim blonde-haired girl, her friend looked at me and said in the same accent, "Hi-ya, it's my birthday today and we're having a bit of a celebration. Are you going to give us a kiss then?"

Amused and slightly embarrassed I leant forward and in a gentlemanly fashion, kissed her on the cheek. Her friend glanced at me and smiled; I returned the compliment. They took their drinks and sat down at a table near the bar. The music was loud and the club was buzzing. As the evening went on, I kept glancing over to the blonde-haired girl. She and her dark-haired friend were now sitting with a colleague of mine called Malcolm, I though this would be a good time to move over. There was a spare seat between them.

"Hi, you don't mind if I join you, do you?" I said as nonchalantly as I could.

"No, not at all," she replied.

"My name's Don, what's yours?"

I couldn't hear her reply. "What?" I said above the din.

"It's Christine."

"Hi, it's nice to meet you."

"Same here," she answered. "Sorry, what did you say your name was?"

"Don'll do," I said.

"What? *Donelldo*?"

"Yes, it's Italian," I said, picking up on her misunderstanding and hoping to turn it to my advantage. "My surname is Lucey."

"What a strange name…"

The noise of the music gave me the opportunity to move closer to her. She looked at me suspiciously. "How can you get away with your hair being so long?" she asked.

I was lucky. As a Physical Training Instructor I had a trade, allowing me to wear an army-issue PTI tracksuit. I rarely attended daily parades and seldom came under the scrutiny of the company sergeant major. As a result I could grow my hair slightly longer than most. I rather looked like the civilians who used to frequent the many clubs and different units on the Tidworth camp.

It was getting late but I soon discovered that Christine and her friends were nurses stationed at the garrison military hospital. They lived in Nightingale Lodge, accommodation for single female personnel. It was a section of the camp totally and unequivocally out of bounds to us men.

Eventually the music stopped and the dim disco lighting was abruptly replaced by the glare of the bright, fluorescent barrack-room lights. The draped silky parachute material, which earlier had added softness and sensuality to the converted room, now appeared drab and meaningless. Only a few people had remained to the end to brave the reality of these stark surroundings! I was wishing that the magic of the evening could have lasted all night. I plucked up my courage and asked Christine if I could walk her home. She agreed. Accompanied by her friends, we strolled back to the Lodge.

When we were finally alone, we managed to talk quietly for a short while before the duty corporal, who would later become our good friend, beckoned her inside. I left feeling happy and contented. I had never bothered much about a steady relationship before. When I was seventeen, a girlfriend had persuaded me to stay at her home one night for her eighteenth birthday celebrations. The party had lasted all night. I missed my train back to barracks the following day, arrived late for parade and was confined to camp for fourteen days as punishment. Girlfriends and parties had generally been my downfall through my teens. Neither seemed compatible with an army career. I was more of an action man, occasionally socialising with the boys.

But now I was smitten, if somewhat apprehensive. Did she like me? She had certainly been friendly enough, a little reserved, but that was a good thing. Then a nagging doubt crept over me. Why on earth did I say my name was *Donelldo*? I felt a shudder of embarrassment. I had met this wonderful and intelligent girl, who was probably nineteen or twenty years old and was a qualified nurse. I had never been out with anyone who matched her charm and beauty. Her hair was long, soft and golden, reaching down to her waist. She spoke in a gentle manner and was so full of fun. I wanted to see her again. Yet all I had said was goodbye and I hadn't even kissed her.

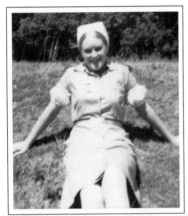

Christine, 1976

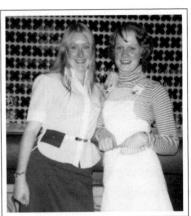

Christine and friend, Jane, at the club where we met, 1976

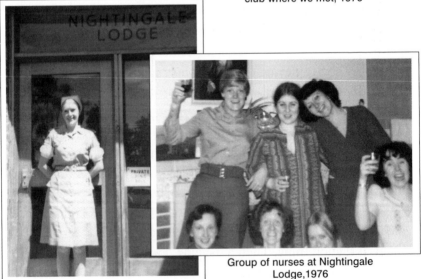

Christine at Nightingale Lodge, Tidworth,

Group of nurses at Nightingale Lodge, 1976

TWO

I felt like the luckiest guy in the world

My first date with Christine was an unmitigated disaster. On the Saturday morning of October 23, 1976, I had decided to stroll towards Nightingale Lodge in the hope of being able to see Christine again. When I arrived, I was confronted by a large red and white military sign on the perimeter gate, instructing: PLEASE RING BELL FOR ATTENTION. The gate was quite a distance from the main door of the one-storey building, which was surrounded by wooden fencing four metres high. I might as well be stuck in the middle of Salisbury Plain. How on earth were they going to hear me ringing the bell?

Should I go in anyway? Perhaps not. These premises were out of bounds to me and I did not want to get Chris into any trouble. I had no reasonable excuse for being there.

I had just started to walk away when a voice called out, "Can I help you?"

I turned to find a uniformed, dark-haired young woman standing a little way off on the other side of the gate. She was staring at me.

"Y… Yes," I stammered, "I'm looking for Christine, she's a nurse. We met last night at the Medic's Club."

"There's no one here but me," she informed me. "I think you must mean Private Hague. She's gone into Salisbury, shopping. Can I give her a message when she gets back?"

"Um… No, it's OK – I'll pop back later. You can tell her Don called, just to say hello. What's your name?" I asked.

"I'm Corporal Derrick," she said crisply, still studying me from behind the gate.

"Right. OK. Thanks." As there was nothing more I could do, I said goodbye and wandered off.

When I returned later in the day Christine and I arranged to see each other that evening and I arrived to collect her. My recollection, when I first caught sight of her, waiting for me by the gates of Nightingale Lodge, is that she looked absolutely stunning. I can still remember what she was wearing: a red knee-length skirt with a blue-and-white striped blouse, a red choker with a gold pendant and a gold-bracelet watch, which was a twenty-first birthday present from her parents. Christine was five foot eight inches tall and her full-length black leather coat complemented her height.

I felt like the luckiest guy in the world.

She asked tentatively where we were going: I told her it was a surprise. I had arranged for a friend to take us into Salisbury. We walked over to the Officers' Mess to meet him. Matt Fenwick, a new recruit to the unit, was standing at the bar with a number of other officers fresh out of Sandhurst. "Hello," he called out, beckoning us over to join him. "Fancy a drink?"

I assured Chris that we would not stay long and told her that Matt had offered to drive us to Salisbury; I promised her that we would be there by eight-thirty. Time went on and Matt insisted that we have another drink.

"Just one more then, Matt," I said, not wishing to offend him. Chris settled for a coffee. I could see that she was looking bored and I felt a little agitated. After all, it was our first date. I interrupted Matt and reminded him about our lift, before he got carried away to the point of having one drink too many. It was already getting late and Chris had to be back at Nightingale Lodge before midnight.

Matt finished his drink and we made our way out to his car, a light blue Mini-Coupé. As we drove away I was beginning to wonder if this was such a good idea after all. I had always felt uncomfortable in small cars. I sat in the front and Christine sat in the back. We approached the main A303 road with the radio blaring loud music.

I knew that Matt had had a couple of drinks but this didn't seem excessive. I assumed he was still capable of driving. I didn't drive at that time, and there weren't the strict drink-driving laws that we have today.

It was a dismal evening and very foggy. We turned out of a junction to join the main road. Suddenly there was a loud bang and the car shuddered. We had been hit by another vehicle. Our car careered sideways across the road, the sound of metal scraping on concrete screeching in my ears. We came to a standstill; battered, shaken and pushed up against the kerbside. A pungent smell of petrol fumes was filling the car. For a moment everything was totally still. The sound of the loud music on the radio was eerie in the stillness.

I was lying sideways, against the passenger door. Nobody wore seat belts then. Matt held onto the steering wheel, leaning against me. I looked around to check if Chris was all right. We were in total darkness, disorientated and scared to hell. None of us were able to move. I tried to get out but it was impossible. Chris was lying still. Matt was trapped by his door, which had been hit and crushed inwards. I could hear shouting outside.

Suddenly the car began to move. A group of soldiers had stopped nearby and scrambled out of their military vehicle. They were physically pulling the car upright. Our rescuers freed all of us, helping us to climb out one by one. What a good feeling it was to be on the outside, looking at the mangled Mini. Chris, although slightly shocked, was amazingly calm. A military Land Rover took us to a nearby Officers' Mess and then back to our own garrison.

None of us had any apparent injuries but later that evening Chris complained of head and neck pain and decided to go to the garrison hospital for a check-up. She had sustained a whiplash injury and was kept in overnight for observations. When I called the next day to see her, she was sitting up in bed reading the Sunday papers.

Embarrassed, I apologised profusely for the previous evening and promised to take her out again if she would let me, assuring her that this time we would stick to public transport. She agreed.

Fortunately she was feeling better and began telling me about a NCO's course she would attend in a few weeks. This was good news. She had only been in the service a short time and already she was on her way to being promoted. Chris had all the right attributes to supervise junior ranks; she was well-educated and had a confident and charming personality. I was immensely relieved that she did not blame me about the way our first date had turned out. We arranged to meet when she was feeling better.

Matt was not so lucky. He appeared before the Commanding Officer on Monday morning, was severely reprimanded and was on his way to Germany by three o'clock the following day. I think he achieved the accolade of having served the shortest time ever with the unit and possibly he had the quickest posting in the British Army!

A few days later I called to see Chris at Nightingale Lodge, armed with a box of chocolates and a small present that Matt had asked me to give her. Chris opened Matt's gift to find a pair of gold earrings. Before I had the chance to explain that they were an apology from Matt, she kissed my cheek as a small token of appreciation. I swiftly moved on to tell her that Matt had been posted. I think we both guessed the real reason and our suspicions were later confirmed. We heard that he had admitted to having consumed more than a couple of gin and tonics that night. It was some years before I eventually confessed to Chris that the earrings were from Matt. And Christine, being Christine, just laughed.

That's how gracious she was.

We saw each other quite frequently during the weeks leading up to Christmas. Chris had passed the three-week residential course at the training depot in Aldershot and gained promotion to the rank of corporal.

One day we went to Bristol to visit my mother with our friend, Mary Derrick, the duty corporal that I had met the first time I went to Nightingale Lodge. My mum liked them both and was curious to know which of the two women was my girlfriend. I resolved to keep her in suspense for a while.

*

On New Year's Eve I went by train to Durham, Chris's hometown, to meet her family. I had completed my guard duty and now sported a new hairstyle: short back and sides, the regulation army haircut. The Company Sergeant Major had previously copped me and asked me 'nicely' to make an appointment with the barber. It was somewhat ironic that I should now look more like a soldier just as I was about to start my leave.

Chris met me at the station. This was my first visit to the northeast of England, and it was an eye opener. We started celebrating the New Year festivities in the northern way by accompanying her parents to a nearby public house. Here we met some of Chris's friends, ex-school chums and nurses with whom she had trained at the local hospital. I had never encountered such hospitality or friendliness before. Northern people have a natural ability to make you feel welcomed. Almost immediately everyone talks to you as if they have known you all of their life. I felt like a member of the community after only a few hours.

Now I understood the secret of Christine's personality and character. Northerners differ from southerners, who tend to be more reserved and less sociable. Almost every home I visited boasted a roaring coal fire; helping these hardy northerners to ward off the severity of their winters and adding to their cheery welcome. Chris was the eldest of five, with two younger brothers and two younger sisters. Her parents, John and Cicily, were both local residents born in Durham; they had lived in the north all their lives. Her father was an engineer. Chris had obtained secretarial qualifications in the early 1970's. Shortly afterwards she qualified as a state enrolled nurse, before leaving home to join the army as a nurse at the beginning of 1976.

Christine's parents lived in Brandon, a small village six miles from Durham. Their large semi-detached house, surrounded by other well-kept, privately owned and council properties, lay in a grid of small villages within the heavily populated suburban sprawl of County Durham. This backdrop of rural life nestled unseen, lost in the maze of major roads that led to other imposing northern cities, such as Newcastle and Gateshead.

*

At the end of a delightful visit it was time for us to return to Tidworth; back to military life. A New Year and a new beginning in our lives. We sat close to each other, holding hands on the train travelling south, both knowing that we were hopelessly in love. The rocking motion and rhythm of the train had made Chris drowsy and she moved closer, resting her head gently on my shoulder. I placed my arm around her and stroked her beautiful long hair reassuringly; she sighed happily and then closed her eyes, gradually falling asleep. I could not remember ever feeling happier.

Ten or fifteen minutes later the ticket collector shattered our peaceful interlude and I was forced to rummage awkwardly through my pockets in the search for the tickets, awakening Chris in the process. He gave us one of those 'knowing looks' as he made his way up the aisle. Chris and I couldn't help grinning inanely at each other, half-pleased and half-embarrassed.

For the rest of the journey we talked about our ambitions in life and, more importantly, of our prospects for a long-term relationship and future plans. Chris was happy with her career as a nurse and had no aspirations to travel abroad as a service woman. She wanted to further her career and promotional prospects but she was not overly excited about military life. I was soon due to finish my army service and become a civilian again.

*

Six weeks later, on St Valentine's Day, 1977, I spent my last day in the army, having completed nine years of service. I went back to my mother's home in Bristol. It seemed like only yesterday that Chris and I had been sitting on the train talking about our plans for the future. Now here I was, sitting on another train, leaving behind so many memories of service life, leaving behind my friends, my colleagues and Christine. We had said our goodbyes the night before and had promised to phone each other and to write.

For the next three months we spoke regularly on the phone and saw each other on occasional weekends. One evening during April Chris told me the surprising news that most of the units at Tidworth, including the garrison hospital, were closing down and amalgamating with other military units in Aldershot, well-known as a very regimental garrison town. The soldiers stationed at Tidworth had been used to a more relaxed working environment and I felt sorry for those who had to move. It seemed that I had chosen the right time to end my army career.

Chris was posted to the family medical centre at the RAF Hospital, Wroughton, near Swindon. I soon found employment in civilian life, working for a small electrical engineering company, a family business. I earned a good salary, my hair started to grow again and I was feeling great. I was happy to be back with my family again. It was springtime and the new lifestyle was definitely agreeing with me. It was not going to remain that way for long.

THREE

A new life together

Chris had settled into her new posting. Built in 1939 and once known as the RAF General Hospital, the Princess Alexandra's Hospital, Wroughton, was now sharing its role with army and naval medical personnel. Most of the single servicemen and women stayed in military accommodation near the hospital but they had the option of 'living out'. After the first few weeks, Chris and her friend, Joyce, decided to find rented accommodation and they moved into a three-bedroom semi-detached house in the village of Wroughton. Soon afterwards I received a letter from Chris. It was clear that she wanted me to move in with them and share the expenditure. At that time the rent was sixty-five pounds a month.

Everything was going well for me in Bristol. I was happy with my employment and had been accepted into the team. When I broke the news that I was thinking of moving to Wiltshire my employers offered me a salary rise. I was also close to the family, especially to their ten-year-old daughter, Philippa, who often rushed in to see me at the factory on her way home from school.

Every now and again I would daydream; thinking of how much Chris and I would enjoy having a son or daughter. Chris often mentioned that she would like to have a baby one day. Knowing Philippa for several weeks had given me an insight into the mind of this little girl. In later years it was to help me enormously in understanding my own daughter, Rebecca.

It was a difficult decision to make, but I had decided to leave my job. On my last day at work I waited to say goodbye to Philippa. I felt guilty that I would not be there any more to talk to her after school. These chats had made her so happy. She cried and begged me not to go. I promised to write every day and to visit as often as I could.

On a warm evening one Friday in the summer of 1977 I arrived at 37 Saville Crescent, Wroughton. When Chris opened the door and threw her arms around me in a passionate embrace, I instantly knew that I had made the right decision. This was to be our home for the next eighteen months. Later that year Joyce moved out when she was posted to Hong Kong.

During the latter part of that year Chris, herself, was admitted to Princess Alexandra's Hospital for a minor operation to remove a cyst from her left wrist. She was about to encounter a foretaste of the sort of medical negligence that was later to change our entire lives. The cyst was removed successfully without any complications, but she returned home with a white rectangular patch covering her left eye. She told me there had been a slight 'accident' in the operating theatre. A technician had accidentally dropped an instrument on her eye during the surgery.

Chris told me this without malice or emotion. I could not understand her calm approach. When I pointed out that she might have been seriously injured, she simply said, "Don't worry, I'll be fine," and left it at that. This forgiving way was so typical of Chris.

It was not my way, however. A few days later when the patch was removed, my cynicism led me to deliver a few critical remarks to Chris, concerning the 'professionalism' of the theatre technician. These remarks just washed over Chris.

She returned to work and for a while the incident was the talk of the hospital, causing much embarrassment for the young theatre nurse. For Chris, it was a minor accident, just one of those things. "Could happen to anyone," she said.

One day I returned home to find Chris and an entourage of girlfriends sitting on the lounge floor drinking tea and browsing excitedly through an assortment of glossy magazines. Guessing they were choosing winter outfits and thinking this was a good time to go out for a run, I tactfully left them to enjoy themselves. As I got ready, I could hear occasional words: *"wedding… guests…*

honeymoon?" I pondered on this as I jogged, wondering about whom they were talking. We had discussed marriage… but… no, Chris would have said something to me, surely…?

I got back about an hour later and immediately noticed the same pile of magazines on the coffee table. Her friends had gone but Chris was still very excited. She had prepared a hot bath for me with essential oils and candles around the room. I was left to luxuriate in the bath with a tall glass of claret. It was obvious there was something she wanted to tell me.

When I emerged Chris coaxed me to sit down beside her on the sofa. I soon discovered the reason for all of the pampering. Today we were going to talk 'seriously' about our wedding plans, I was told. We did exactly that for the next few hours. Before long we had provisionally drawn them up. We were to marry in the summer of 1978. Chris wanted a white wedding, with plenty of guests, a large cake and an exotic honeymoon abroad. It was to be the archetypal wedding, every couple's dream. By the end of our lovely romantic evening we had planned our future, agreed to build a home together and to enjoy our married life for a while before starting a family.

We became engaged shortly before Christmas. I remember getting an advance on my pay as we were paid weekly in those days in order to buy the diamond and sapphire ring.

So much had happened in just under a year.

It was now the start of the New Year and the January sales were in full swing. We resisted the temptation to spend money and kept our savings for our special day. The wedding date had been officially booked and Chris was designing and making her own gown, as well as the bridesmaids' dresses. She enjoyed planning things and had an innate ability to organise without being overpowering.

At last, after several months of dressmaking, I picked up the final pin from the floor, not wanting ever to see another in my life. Still, looking at the end result made me feel so proud to be marrying such a talented person.

On the morning of Saturday, 22 July, 1978, our wedding day, I awoke feeling the worst for wear after the customary stag party the night before. It had seemed bizarre being separated from Chris that night; keeping with the tradition of not seeing the bride before the ceremony. That day I felt strangely apprehensive as the hours drew closer to meeting her in the church, even though we had already shared twelve months of our lives together.

The wedding took place in Durham, which seemed appropriate, as this was the city where Chris had grown up and most of her family and friends still lived there. The small group on my side of the family had travelled from the south. They were all in awe of the beauty of County Durham.

This was indeed the perfect place to get married. The old, disused mining communities are apparent everywhere. Villages near Chris's parents' home, such as Langley Moor, Meadowfield and Brancepeth, are distinguished by their own distinct characters. The early nineteenth century terraced houses, bellowing smoke from their chimney pots, seemed frozen in time. Neville's Cross, the site of a famous battle in Cromwell's time was situated nearby; other famous landmarks included the historic Durham Cathedral, the infamous Durham Reformatory and Durham University.

As a young child Chris had been a member of the Boyne Corp, a division of the Salvation Army and often received book prizes for her good conduct, diligence, and regular attendance. Her collection of awards dated back to December, 1963, when she was eight years old. This was an important facet of her childhood. She was often encouraged by her parents to help others, in particular, the poor and the elderly. These traits continued as she grew into a young woman and throughout the rest of her life.

We were married in a Salvation Army Church in Meadowfield. It was a beautiful white wedding. The three bridesmaids, my sister,

Ann, and Chris's two younger sisters, Pauline and Janet, wore elegantly designed turquoise gowns with glittering gold speckles, the results of Chris's skilful handiwork. Chris's sister, Pauline, caught the bride's bouquet.

We sat outside the church for initial photographs and then moved to a local park for more. That evening we left our guests enjoying the reception as we slipped quietly away to spend the first night of our honeymoon in a small country hotel near Durham.

The following day we were on our way to Jersey, not the exotic honeymoon location we had originally planned but the next best thing. We loved the English/French ambience of Jersey, its eclectic mixture of restaurants and the plethora of exclusive shops selling elegant jewellery and other quality goods, all at duty free prices. The scenery of the island appealed to us enormously, as did the warmth and friendliness of the local people. They still live with the grim reminder of German occupation during the last war, as evidenced by places such as the German underground hospital in the province of St Lawrence.

We were particularly impressed by the Battle of the Flowers Parade, an annual event in which a convoy of vehicles and trailers bearing the most spectacular, aromatic floral displays moves in slow procession along promenade and main thoroughfare of St Helier. Enthusiastic crowds thronged the pavements to applaud layers of carnations, the island's most popular flower, bouquets of romantic red and white roses, multitudes of orchids and birds of paradise and huge quantities of chrysanthemums. Chris, a keen fan of the popular television show, *Coronation Street*, was delighted to see Ken Barlow the actor, William Roach, aboard one float, sitting beside Miss Jersey.

Alas, our fourteen days soon passed and we returned home with fond memories of the island. We promised ourselves that we would return in the near future, bringing our families to see the sights. It was a promise that we never kept.

Chris completed her short-term service in the Queen Alexandra's Royal Army Nursing Corp soon after our honeymoon and she then became a civilian. Female service employees had two options upon marriage, they could either continue their employment or they were able to resign, regardless of how much or little time they had been employed. By contrast, male soldiers either had to complete their contracts, which could be anything from three to twenty-two years of service, or they could obtain 'Discharge by Purchase' which meant paying a sum to end the contract.

I knew that Chris was glad to have left the service, but felt that she might miss some of the camaraderie that came with military life. What mattered most, though, was the sense of freedom that we both experienced. No more duties to worry about, no longer having to fear separation due to training courses. I was also very glad not to have to press any more uniforms, a task for which I had inadvertently volunteered, as part of sharing the household chores!

Chris paid regular visits to the family planning clinic. She cared about her health and knew how important it was to have medical examinations, most importantly, cervical smear checks. She explained the process to me once and described how a doctor or nurse took an internal swab from the cervix to obtain cells for culture in the laboratory and for investigation. There was no embarrassment between us about discussing this or any other feminine issue.

Chris had been using an oral contraceptive pill from the age of twenty, having suffered previously with painful periods. The particular brand she used was effective with no notable side effects and it suited us, since starting a family was not a priority at this stage of our marriage

In August we bought our first house, a suburban terraced dwelling with three bedrooms, located close to a busy road, which was the main route into Swindon. It was an old property in need of repair and we spent several months renovating the exterior and redecorating the rooms. I didn't think that my DIY skills were very good, but I surprised myself by managing to build a Cotswold stone fireplace. This impressed Chris but it was my only claim to fame as an amateur interior designer.

Both Chris and I were career-minded. I worked for a dairy company and Chris started a new job as a care assistant, looking after the elderly at Langton House in Wroughton, a purpose-built local authority home for sixty-three residents. After a year, we sold our home in Swindon, made a slight profit and moved to a semi-detached house in the village of Hilmarton, in rural Wiltshire, where I was able to continue indulging my passion for outdoor exercise.

I would often run to work in Swindon, a distance of eleven miles. At the end of my shift I would cycle home, alternating daily between the inward and outward means of transport. This was good training for my next event. I had entered my first sponsored marathon, to raise money for the Residents' Amenities Fund at Langton House. Much of our spare time was dedicated to voluntary work and I became involved in practically every event that Langton House organised. All of the money raised went towards making the home more comfortable for the residents, enabling them to purchase essential equipment and a new electronic organ for their entertainment. Terry Collier, the Officer-in-Charge, often played for them on a regular basis.

In June, 1980, Chris was promoted to Deputy Officer-in-Charge of Langton House, and a party was organised to celebrate the occasion. I was very proud of her. She had worked so hard and had achieved so much in such a short time. The next step would be to gain further promotion and eventually become an Officer-in-Charge of one of the Wiltshire County Council residential homes for the elderly.

At first I was a little sceptical about homes for old people in our society. I thought that the people living in them were soon forgotten by their immediate families and lived out the rest of their lives lonely and unhappy. Seeing, at first hand, how they were cared for changed my opinion. The residents enjoyed a wide variety of social gatherings and celebrations. What I enjoyed most about these incredible elderly people was their ability to keep their independence, something that Chris felt strongly about and always encouraged. She was fond of everyone in her care and she showed no favouritism.

Bereavement at the home had the biggest impact on the staff and residents, but somehow they just accepted this and continued with daily life. They were true professionals, every one of them.

FOUR

No alarm bells were ringing

We were extremely happy during the early years of our marriage. We had an abundance of friends, a good social life and spent many wonderful times planning and building our lives together, as well as enjoying holidays both abroad and in the UK.

Both of us also enjoyed excellent health. I was hardly ever ill and would only visit my doctor if I had a particularly bad cold or something similarly minor. More often than not I only wanted a touch of sympathy. I pursued my fitness regime, competing in running events up and down the country, from Devon to Newcastle, raising sponsorship money for the Residents' Amenities Fund at Langton House. I would eventually complete fifteen full marathons, numerous half-marathons and a variety of other middle-distance races.

Like many young women, Chris looked after her health. In particular, she guarded against the serious illnesses that can affect young women and their ability to have children. Being a qualified nurse, she knew the statistical risks of cancer. She had regular check-ups, including cervical smear tests. In taking care of her health she did, like most of us, rely on the advice given to her by her GP, the local hospital and the family planning clinic.

During this time there were, of course, no alarm bells ringing to alert either of us to any serious concern about the smear-testing capabilities of the medical fraternity. The negative smear test results Chris received were always reassuring. These tests were carried out at first during Chris's army service and then while she was stationed at the RAF hospital. The results were analysed by the Cytology Department in the local Princess Margaret Hospital (PMH). Like all patients, Chris was never informed of the exact wording in her smear results, she was simply told every time that they were either 'clear' or 'negative'. We were to find out very much later that, in fact, the wording on most of the smear reports described abnormalities in the cells which, at the very least indicated that further testing should have been done within a short time. The results of Chris's smear tests in the decade between 1977 and 1988 have been summarised by Pathologist Professor Roger Cotton, and are presented on page 188.

Almost all of Chris's smear tests, including the first one taken in 1977, should have given medical staff cause for concern; most of them, one in 1978, two in 1986 and one in 1988, indicated immediate gynaecological referral. No smears were taken at all between 1983 and 1986. I am convinced that events would have turned out very differently if someone had been more thorough in acting on the information that was available from a very early stage.

But we were unaware of any problem and we were concentrating on our career development. I had recently been promoted and Chris was well into her role as Deputy Officer-in-Charge of homes for the elderly at Wiltshire County Council. On 22 January, 1982, something happened that could have changed the course of my life. At 5:30 that morning I was on my way to work, driving alone and travelling at sixty miles an hour. As I approached a sharp bend in the road I hit a patch of black ice and lost control. Everything happened 'quickly-yet-slowly'. There were a few lost seconds, the sensation of turning over and over, a sudden explosion of noise, followed by the inevitable silence. The car had come to rest at last, facing across a frost-covered field; it was a total write-off but I was uninjured. Chris was so relieved that I had been wearing my seat belt, something she had nagged me about incessantly, ever since the accident on our first date. Her advice had probably saved my life. Once again I had managed to cheat death; someone 'up there' seemed to be watching over us.

But in October of that year Chris fell seriously ill for the first time. She was experiencing excruciating abdominal pains and was referred by her local GP to Princess Alexandra's Hospital where she had served as an army nurse, for further tests. It was here that she met Group Captain Baxendall, the consultant gynaecologist, for the first time. I remember him well: a tall, middle-aged man of medium-build, balding, who wore his long white coat like a badge of office over his RAF uniform. He was well-respected, perhaps even slightly feared by his subordinates, who worked alongside him with a certain amount of caution. Chris thought he was somewhat abrupt but commented that she thought his bark was worse than his bite. Naturally, she put her faith in his professionalism as a doctor.

Dr Baxendall examined Chris in the hospital clinic, adjacent to Ward One where gynaecology and ante/postnatal patients had their beds. This was his domain and nobody dared step on his toes. He could find no abnormalities during the examination but as Chris's medical records showed that she had had salpingitis, an inflammation of the fallopian tubes, in 1977, another appointment was arranged for November.

On 28 November, Dr. Baxendall performed a laparoscopy, an incision in the abdomen wall enabling him to investigate the abdominal organs. He confirmed that Chris had a reoccurrence of salpingitis and he prescribed antibiotics.

In a follow-up appointment in January, 1983, he diagnosed endometriosis, a condition in which endometrial, tissue lining of the womb, occurs in other sites. Chris was given medication to ease her pain.

By February the pain had lessened and Dr Baxendall suggested that she could take the oral contraceptive pill, Eugynon 30, as an alternative to the antibiotics until she wanted to become pregnant. By May, 1983, Chris was symptom-free and Dr. Baxendall made no further arrangements to see her.

Chris stopped taking the pill in October, 1983. We had decided that the time was right to start a family. Nine months later, on 3 July 1984, our GP wrote to Dr Baxendall informing him that Chris was pregnant and should be booked into the hospital for delivery. Subsequent visits to the clinic continued to monitor her progress.

That year I completed another marathon: my first London entry. I managed to finish in three hours, eleven minutes. Chris was there to support me again but she fell asleep in the car on the way home, apparently exhausted after following my progress at the different vantage points around the twenty-six mile course.

Chris and I looked forward to having a baby. We had been further reassured by Chris's GP that the results of smear test results obtained during the previous three years, were all reported as 'clear' and/or 'negative'. It was an exciting time for us. We thought that Chris's health problems were over and were simply looking forward to the baby. Chris was ecstatic. Soon we would have a child of our own.

*

On 13 July Chris was admitted to the Princess Alexandra Hospital with light vaginal bleeding and our happy news was soon replaced by disappointment. An ultrasound scan and pregnancy test showed no evidence of pregnancy; Chris had miscarried after thirteen weeks of gestation. This was a traumatic and difficult time. I will never forget the look in Chris's eyes as the sense of her loss gripped her. No longer the bright-eyed mother-to-be, she was obviously deeply mourning the loss of our baby. The stage of development that the baby had reached was not equal to the depth of her grief.

After leaving hospital on 17 July, Chris suffered another episode of vaginal bleeding. It lasted for several weeks and gave us further cause for concern. No medical explanation was given to us for the miscarriage and I could not understand the reluctance of her doctors to provide Chris with feasible answers to help her come to terms with what had happened, nor did she receive any form of counselling.

Chris was very distressed and we talked about why she had been put through such an ordeal. I suggested that it was God's way of preventing something from happening that was not right. Perhaps it had somehow better prepared her body to conceive a child in the near future. Although I was not as religiously minded as she was, I found this explanation appropriate at the time and Chris seemed to accept my reasoning. "Perhaps you're right, Don," she said, "maybe these things are just meant to be."

But she sounded small and lost when she said it and I was crying for her inwardly.

Although I hadn't suffered the physical loss that Chris had, I shared the mental and emotional distress. I arranged a weekend break in the tiny fishing village of Looe in Cornwall, hoping that it would help Chris to get over the ordeal.

Gradually we did manage to put aside our loss; we buoyed ourselves up with the thought that we could always try again.

*

It was not long before the 'itchy feet syndrome' returned and we began house hunting. A new estate was being built on the outskirts of Swindon, in the area known as West Swindon: the development was due for completion in the early part of 1985. This area appealed to Chris. She was looking for a four-bedroom detached house. I was anxious about her ambitious ideas and asked her if she was sure we could afford it. Were we doing the 'right thing,' all the usual uncertainties that men will utter when they do not see the need for change. Chris's answer was that we could manage, if we were prepared to work harder and save more. Hmm... a brand new house meant new carpets and curtains, new furniture and... well, practically new everything. I thought it all rather daunting but went along with it.

We moved into our new home on 5 May, 1985. As it happened, it was lucky that we moved when we did: shortly afterwards, our former neighbours' home was destroyed by fire, causing extensive damage to our old house.

Chris began to put her creative skills into action and soon our new home began taking shape. Occasionally we had disagreements about the over-expenditure of our monthly budget, but doesn't everyone? I have to confess that I didn't help much with cutting back, I yielded to temptation and agreed to purchase a leather chesterfield and saddleback chair!

Neither Chris nor I was afraid of extra hard work. In February Chris had completed a special unit assignment, a demanding two-year non-residential course and had gained a qualification for a Certificate in Social Services (CCS) for the care of elderly people.

It was not long before we started to wonder whether it might be a good idea to look into owning our own residential home for the elderly. Our search for a suitable place took precedence over other matters. Chris was qualified to manage such a business, I would continue my own career, giving occasional help when it was needed.

Eventually we found the ideal property, Norbury House, in a quiet little village called Purton, three miles from our own home. It was in need of a little repair but it had potential. We soon organised everything that had to be done, making sure that we complied with Wiltshire Social Services regulations on managing a residential home. All that remained was the final confirmation on the finance to buy the property. This seemed imminent and had already been agreed in principle. The owners had previously accepted our offer and all appeared to be well.

We thought that nothing could go wrong but it did. Four days before exchanging contracts, we were gazumped. Someone else offered the vendors more money and they accepted. We were both devastated and were on the verge of losing our faith in human nature.

Determined to continue we began looking at other properties, though I think that the disappointment had dampened Chris's enthusiasm for the venture. However, we were to find out that one of my mother's old sayings, that good things can come out of bad, would later prove true.

In January, 1986, Chris had a smear test taken by her GP. She was later informed that it was clear. Dr Baxendall saw her again in March. By this time she was becoming worried over her infertility; eighteen months had passed since her miscarriage. Dr Baxendall thought that her problem was related to irregular ovulation and he prescribed Provera to induce withdrawal bleeding and Clomid, the trade name for clomiphene, which is used to stimulate the ovaries to produce eggs. It was arranged that I should also have a sperm count.

Chris subsequently had two periods at thirty-three-day intervals. At her appointment at the Gynaecology Clinic on 28 April the same Clomid dosage was recommended for a further four months. My sperm count proved to be normal. Chris was due to return to the clinic again in June, after we had a short holiday with her family in Durham.

One night, while we were staying with her parents, something frightening happened. Chris began clutching at her abdomen and complaining of severe pains. These had started in a mild enough fashion a few hours earlier but had continued to increase in intensity. It was now three o'clock in the morning. There was no time to call out a doctor The only alternative was to get her to Dryburn Hospital as quickly as possible. The hospital doctor's immediate diagnosis was that she was displaying the symptoms of an ectopic pregnancy, one occurring outside the womb.

However, after several hours in the operating theatre, surgeons carried out an emergency operation to remove a cyst from the right ovary. It had ruptured, causing internal bleeding and one of Chris's fallopian tubes had to be removed. The removal of both would, of course, have caused permanent sterilisation.

The surgeon who carried out the operation told us that the cyst was probably caused by a reaction to Clomid. Fortunately it had not caused any further internal complications. After a three-month break from work, Chris returned for her appointment with the gynaecologist. He was aware of her operation and agreed that it had been an unfortunate reaction, but said that she could continue with the course of Clomid, when she was 'fit and well'. Following the experience in Durham, we decided to wait for three months before Chris continued with the fertility drug. A smear test carried out in August, along with the results of previous tests, were reported to Chris as 'negative'. By late October Chris was despondent, feeling that she would never conceive. We discussed the possibility of *in vitro* fertilisation, a test tube baby, but we took no immediate action.

Other aspects of life improved a little. In February, 1987, Chris was promoted to Officer-in-Charge of homes for the elderly at Wiltshire County Council. She was also one of the youngest employees to hold that position in Wiltshire's Social Services Department and, apparently, in the country. She seemed destined for an exciting career, and I was extremely proud of her. Ironically, her new post was in the village of Purton, at a purpose-built home for the elderly, accommodating fifty residents in single bed-sitting rooms. The residents would receive care tailored to their personal needs, and would retain a high degree of self-identity, which was what Chris had always encouraged. The position was ideal for her.

The building, *The Cedars*, was nearing completion and would be ready to open in July. Chris would have the responsibility of organising everything, from the interior decorating, to interviewing and employing twenty new staff, as well as selecting residents from other homes.

A party organised by the staff and residents at Langton House served a twofold purpose: to celebrate Chris's promotion and to wish her farewell. She had spent the past nine years there and everyone would miss her.

In early May, 1987, we received incredibly good news. At last Chris was pregnant. We were jubilant! Naturally we were also quite nervous. With a tinge of scepticism, Chris began the delicate routine of attending the antenatal clinic once more. It was very early days, but she frequented the sessions at the clinic more frequently than most of the other mothers-to-be.

FIVE

The cervix felt 'woody'

The bleeding started again in the thirteenth week of Chris's pregnancy. The symptoms were exactly the same as those preceding the 1984 miscarriage. Everyone feared the worst. When things go wrong in life, inevitably, one looks for a reason. Some tragedies are more difficult to accept than others. Often life simply does not seem fair, yet each challenge can make the sufferer stronger, if only that person can learn to overcome the trials and tribulations. The events that followed were about to prove this, it would certainly test our ability to cope with the unforeseen.

Chris was admitted to hospital for three days of observation and bed rest. Group Captain Baxendall informed her that she was in a 'high risk' situation, obviously meaning that she might lose the baby. Chris's fears where allayed somewhat when the bleeding eventually stopped. A series of tests and an ultrasound scan showed the baby's development was normal.

Chris was able to come home, though the hospital staff continued to provide excellent antenatal attention. Three weeks before the baby was due they recommended that Chris be admitted to the antenatal ward for precautionary bed rest. Daily foetal monitoring continued, reassuring us of the baby's healthy development. However, several days before the birth she was given some disturbing news. Dr Baxendall had previously carried out an internal examination and he told Chris that there appeared to be something irregular about her cervix. He said that it felt 'woody'. As a result the baby could not be delivered normally. He did not elaborate on *why* he thought it felt this way, nor did he mention any other suspicions that he might have had.

Chris left his office in despair, worried about these findings and the lack of explanation. Her own suspicion was that the 'woody' feeling might be associated with the presence of cancer. But as there was nothing she could do about it, except to put it to the back of her mind, she tried to reassure herself that if there was something *seriously* wrong, Dr Baxendall would definitely have told her; after all,*he* should know, being a consultant gynaecologist.

Chris had been told that, because of the irregularity of the cervix, a Caesarean section was planned for Monday, 1 February. She would be given an epidural for this procedure and a thorough examination of the cervix would be performed at the same time. I was originally 'pencilled in' to be present at the birth.

As we might have expected by now, nothing went according to plan. Early on the Saturday, 30 January, Chris's waters broke. Meconium, the discharge that collects in the intestines of an unborn baby, which is usually released shortly after birth, was present in the water. This alerted a maternity nurse to the possibility of foetal distress. An emergency Caesarean was performed. I was unable to go into the operating theatre because of the change in circumstances, as full anaesthesia was now being administered.

I waited anxiously for news. Chris had been in theatre for quite a while, I was not sure how long. I had lost all track of time. My knowledge about Caesarean section was vague. It seemed that the hospital staff, were deliberately keeping me in suspense, which added to my anxiety.

Shortly after two o'clock in the afternoon, a young maternity nurse appeared in the doorway of Chris's room, holding a small bundle in her arms. She glanced towards me, beaming as though I had won a prize: "It's a girl. Congratulations!" she said, I watched her as she moved towards a washbasin and methodically bathed our daughter.

"How's Chris?" I asked immediately.

"The doctor will be here to see you in a minute," she said, as she passed the baby to me, wrapped in a white, downy towel. Her soft lily-white skin was still crinkled in places, the remarkable temporary imprints left on a baby by being curled tightly inside the mother's womb for so long. I peeped at her tiny fingers and toes, tugging unthinkingly at the digits, the way that every elated new parents does. Our daughter had that distinctive newborn baby smell that merged with the scent of Johnson's baby powder. She cried a little to let everyone know she was safe and well, but she didn't wail and wriggle, like some babies.

I cradled my child in my arms as she sucked and consumed ten millilitres of her first feed. She had stopped crying and was content. A generous tuft of red hair stuck out in fine strands all over her head, still damp and ruffled by the nurse's attempt to dry her. I brushed it flat with my hand to make her look more presentable. After I had been allowed to hold her for a short while, the nurse took her into the maternity ward and placed her, into a transparent cot and covered her with a small pink blanket.

The maternity sister, apologising for the doctor's absence, was left to explain Chris's condition to me in the recovery room. She explained that she was still unconscious from the effects of the anaesthetic but there was nothing to worry about, as this was normal. It would soon wear off. It would take several hours before she regained full consciousness. She added that the baby would be fine until Chris had fully recovered.

Rebecca, as we had already decided to name her, had been born at 2:15 pm, weighing 10lbs 11ozs (4850gms), a rather large and healthy baby girl. Chris had always known how to spring the occasional surprise on me, and this was the best yet.

At seven o'clock on Sunday morning, I walked into Chris's room as she lay holding our baby for the first time. She looked pale and exhausted, but managed a smile. She pointed towards the bedside cabinet: "There's a small present in there for you."

I reached inside and removed a gold crucifix and chain. The note read:

To Daddy,
Thank you for looking after Mummy and me.
Love you lots, baby and Mummy.

xxx

I leant forward and kissed them both. At long last Chris's dream had come true. We were blessed with a beautiful baby.

The maternity ward sister arrived to relay a message from the doctor who had delivered Rebecca. He wanted Chris to be referred to the colposcopy clinic for a cone biopsy. She explained that a colposcope was an instrument used to magnify and photograph the cervix. A cone biopsy was the name of a surgical technique whereby a conical or cylindrical section of the lower part of the cervix is removed for analysis.

Needless to say, Chris was distraught and upset by this news and did not want to discuss it. The ward sister tried to reassure her that everything would be fine but Chris was extremely worried, and consequently had a very restless night. She could not understand why a nurse, and not a doctor, had given this information to her. It was all about professional etiquette. This was what upset her the most. Of course, had the doctor actually come in person, the news would still have had the same impact on her but at least her dignity would have been spared.

Group Captain Baxendall saw her later the next day and they discussed the cone biopsy. He told Chris not to worry, suggesting that the delivery doctor was probably jumping the gun. He said that because Rebecca was such a big baby the irregularity of the cervix could have been due to pressure from her head. He did not consider a biopsy to be necessary. This calmed Chris considerably. It was the sort of news she had hoped for, a benign explanation and it had come from her own gynaecologist. This gave her considerable peace of mind. Surely her gynaecologist's explanation would make the most sense. It no longer mattered how the original message had been relayed. It was just comforting to know that a mistake had been made. Now it was time to put all the worry behind her and start enjoying her baby.

Once again Dr Baxendall had made reference to Rebecca's size, saying that it would not be possible to breast-feed her. Chris smiled to herself and thought otherwise but she made no comment as he walked away. She received after-care treatment from the midwife and by early evening she began breast-feeding Rebecca. There were no further complications and Chris and the baby were soon allowed home. Our family was complete. Nothing could possibly go wrong now.

On 21 March, Chris returned to the postnatal clinic, feeling well and confident. Dr Baxendall carried out an internal examination, followed by a cervical smear, which was later reported to Chris by her GP as negative. He noted that Chris was breast-feeding and that there was no vaginal loss. Her bowels and urinary system were working satisfactorily and the abdominal wound had healed. The cervix showed several inflamed glands but there were no problems with the uterus. Dr Baxendall told Chris that everything was 'back to normal'. She was pleased and relieved, her confidence restored.

Several weeks later, Chris began interviewing for a nanny with the intention of returning to work following her maternity leave. We wanted to employ someone for about twenty hours a week, our work shift patterns would allow us to look after Rebecca for the remaining time. We found the perfect nanny: Jean Callar, a petite, jolly and reasonably fit middle-aged grandmother. She was suitably qualified and later proved to have been a very wise choice. Chris returned to work in May, 1988.

At this time Chris was still unaware of the full contents of the cervical smear test results. All of them had been reported to her by her GP as 'clear' or 'negative' *(see table on page 188)*. As a result she continued to believe that there was nothing seriously wrong with her health. There was no reason she should have thought otherwise. Her confidence and morale were boosted by the positive feedback she received from the medical fraternity. The normal effects of recovering from childbirth, postnatal bleeding and occasional tiredness, she could willingly accept.

Our lives were fulfilled and happy. Who could have hoped for anything better? We had a lovely home, promising careers and a beautiful baby. We had enjoyed a short holiday in Malta and returned fully rejuvenated.

I still had military ambitions and Chris had always been supportive in anything I wanted to do, encouraging me to lead my life to the full. I joined the Territorial Army, 21 SAS (Special Air Service) as a part-time soldier. It was quite ironic that I had left the Army in 1977 and then decided to go back into uniform eleven years later. On each alternate weekend for the next two years, I would attend a rigorous selection process; the fitness regime that followed would prepare me for the strenuous time that lay ahead, in more ways than one.

My training pattern allowed me to spend a lot of time with Chris and Rebecca. Chris used to joke that she was glad I was away some weekends so that she could go shopping with her friends and family. She had never been alone at any time in her life; there was always someone around. Now there was that extra-special someone.

I bought a video camera to film Rebecca's development, something for us both to enjoy in later years. Little did I realise that I would also be recording a different and unimaginable story.

*

Chris became increasingly concerned about her postnatal bleeding and she kept regular appointments at the GP's surgery and the hospital clinic. Consultations with her own doctor usually proved inconclusive and left her feeling confused and totally isolated. The doctor would pat her hand reassuringly and say that no treatment was necessary. He would tell her that the hospital was treating her and they knew what they were doing. The bleeding continued and, as the weeks passed, she became weary and lethargic. She put this down to her busy lifestyle; going out to work, as well as looking after the baby and the house.

Unknown to Chris at the time, the usual correspondence went back and forth between Chris's GP, at the time, Dr Holden, and Dr Baxendall, her gynaecologist. On 2 June, Dr Baxendall wrote to the GP to say that the last smear had been reported as showing some abnormal cells and he requested a repeat. On 21 June a repeat smear was taken and the result was reported to Chris as negative on 27 June. The smear was reported as being very inflammatory and a repeat in one year was suggested. However there was gross misinterpretation, Cancerous cells were present, they were in fact inflammatory. Nor did Chris know the contents of her GP's letter to Dr Baxendall on 11 July, 1988, which read as follows:

This lady, whose smear test I have repeated, has improved in the sense that her smear is now merely inflammatory, which is regarded as negative. A repeat smear has been requested in twelve months time, however she is still getting severe post-coital bleeding, thus I do feel she needs to be seen for this.

Chris did not return to the hospital to see Dr Baxendall at his clinic until 22 August. His examination report recorded that she had had no periods since the birth of Rebecca, and he also noted that she was still experiencing post-coital, and inter-menstrual bleeding. But, having regard to the report from her GP, he noted that her smear was now satisfactory. The GP, Dr Holden, in turn received a letter from Dr Baxendall detailing the results of his examination. It read:

Thank you for asking me to see this lady who complains of post-coital bleeding, She has not had a period since confinement six months ago. I note that her recent smear is satisfactory. On

examination the cervix appears normal and the uterus fully
involuted, her cervix looked healthy, the uterus was retroverted
and the appendages were NAD [normal]. I have asked to see her
again in three months when her periods might have returned; no
further investigations are necessary at present.

Chris was not satisfied with the management of her condition. She had not received any explanation for her symptoms that was convincing enough to allay her anxieties. Yet she seemed to have no alternative but to accept that the bleeding would stop one day. I think she knew she was fooling herself. The probability of cancer was still lurking nervously at the back of her mind. She was caught between a rock and a hard place. Her medical background made it difficult for her to disbelieve the doctors, yet at the same time her worries that the killer disease might be present were escalating.

She would confide this to family and close friends. I would listen sympathetically as she talked of her concerns, often aware of the signs of despair. It was agony to witness the deterioration of this strong-minded young woman. Outwardly she continued to appear calm and in control of her life: generating the image of a happy, radiant mother and loving wife. Inwardly, she was in turmoil. With hindsight it is so easy to understand how Chris accepted the diagnosis of these doctors. Why shouldn't she? Wouldn't any patient have done the same? All she ever wanted to hear was 'All clear' or 'negative', which prevented her from succumbing to panic. Then she would always say, "Thank God, it's not cancer, Don."

I thought she was becoming over-anxious every time she mentioned the word 'cancer', Everyone we knew agreed. No one believed she would ever be at risk of contracting the disease. After all, to most of us, cancer is something that happens to *other* people. My own simplistic view was that cancer was a disease contracted by cigarette smokers or the elderly. I was soon to learn otherwise.

Chris was a non-smoker and had always maintained a healthy diet, eating a diet of fruit and vegetables; she never abused her body. I was the potentially unhealthy one; I lived on junk food.

Rebecca was seven months old, a healthy baby with golden hair and dazzling blue eyes. Her young life was progressing naturally. She was our small miracle, who had survived in her mother's womb through the turmoil of a threatened miscarriage and, as we later discovered, probably the onset of carcinoma of the cervix. She brought so much happiness into our lives, yet this special period and precious bond between mother and child was soon to be broken and lost forever.

Six

Tragically misleading

Chris's ill health had started to affect our relationship. We had not been intimate for nearly a year: not since about the middle of Chris's pregnancy. The complications arising from a second threatened miscarriage had made it sensible to refrain and the miscarriage had been followed by postnatal bleeding, which was often referred to as 'post-coital' bleeding, which finally made sexual intercourse impossible. This was distressing enough for both of us, but little did we then know that the symptoms of Chris's unknown illness would eventually become so severe as to cause totally catastrophic changes to our lives.

One day, an incident occurred that shocked me into realising how serious the bleeding was becoming. It happened on 24 October, 1988. We were on holiday, staying at the quiet Aurapraia Hotel and Apartment Complex in the Portuguese resort of Algarve. Chris was in the bathroom and I could hear her crying. Suddenly she called out, "Oh no! Don, something's wrong, I'm bleeding heavily. I think I need a doctor."

I had been filming Rebecca on the video camera as she edged her way around the kitchen in her baby walker. Immediately, I stopped what I was doing and rushed to telephone to reception, but then Chris came out and told me to wait a while. She looked pale and in shock. Her whole body was shaking.

She sat in a chair near the dining room table and said she would just rest. I made her a cup of tea, while Rebecca looked on as she determinedly carried on pushing herself around the room, uttering innocent 'Mama' sounds and other excited outbursts of baby talk.

I sat down next to Chris and she began to cry again, apologising for causing me alarm and anxiety. I comforted her and said that it didn't matter, but perhaps I should still ask for a doctor to see if there was anything that he could do. She wanted to rest and wait a while longer. Thankfully, a few hours later, she managed to recover somewhat and the bleeding had eased enough to avoid having to call for medical assistance. Chris was embarrassed because of the state in which she had left the bathroom and wanted to go back and tidy it up. I persuaded her not to worry, she should just rest: I told her I would attend to it.

It was only when I went into the bathroom that I realised the extent of what had happened to Chris. She had clearly tried to clean up before she came out. Some of the towels had been used to wipe the blood from the tiled floor. But it was obvious that she had lost about half a litre of blood from the haemorrhage. I now saw enough to fully realise the seriousness of her condition. It brought home the stark reality of her anxiety during the previous ten months.

Thankfully there were no more frightening episodes of excessive blood loss, although the bleeding did continue. We decided to continue with our holiday but when we returned home Chris immediately visited her doctor. He told her she should not worry as she had an appointment at the hospital in four or five weeks time and the matter could wait until then. He added that her haemoglobin level, the iron-containing protein that fills red blood cells, was all right. Nothing could go too seriously wrong.

Her last hospital appointment in November of that year ended as it began ten months earlier. Things remained 'inconclusive'. Chris had continually been told that there was nothing really wrong. The bleeding was simply an unfortunate reaction due to upset hormone levels. Dr Baxendall concluded his findings by saying that the blood loss was caused by a hormonal imbalance brought about by breast-feeding Rebecca. He also stated that he was not concerned because the smear results were clear. But in only two months' time Dr Baxendall and his medical colleagues were to realise that their assumptions and professional judgement had been tragically misleading.

Christmas Day, 1988, was not a traditional white Christmas, but a dry, cold morning with sunshine beaming through the window. Concentrated through the glass, the warmth of its golden rays belied the true chill of the winter outside. Our recent memories of hospitals, doctors and all things medical were temporarily cast from our minds. It was Rebecca's first Christmas. We were together as a family and looking forward to the festivities. Chris was extremely happy, this was a joyous occasion and we were going to make the most of our day.

Laughter and excitement filled the room as we hurriedly opened our presents, the pleasure of watching Rebecca attempting to unwrap the gifts with her tiny fingers adding to the moment. This was how we had always envisaged spending Christmas with our daughter, just as our parents had done with us. It was wonderful to see her so content. Chris sat close to Rebecca and they played with her new toys. I quietly slipped away, leaving them both to enjoy a few special minutes together. Those private moments of closeness between mother and child will be etched in my memory forever. I could never have believed then that this lovely family occasion would be so different in future years.

Chris prepared our Christmas meal in readiness for the arrival of my family, who had been invited to share our day. Later, some friends would visit to join in the celebrations. Since Chris enjoyed the occasion so much that she wanted to share some time with those less fortunate, we spent the latter part of the day with staff and residents at the Cedars Home for the Elderly. Chris had promised to take Rebecca to see them and they seemed to fall in love with our child on sight, her natural boisterousness adding great enjoyment to their Christmas festivities. Only Chris's 'postnatal' bleeding, which still persisted during this time, marred our joy.

January 30, 1989, was Rebecca's first birthday. We had planned a party for the afternoon with two special guests, Rebecca's childminder, Jean and her husband, David. Chris had a hospital appointment that morning. It had been two months since her last visit. Dr Baxendall, who observed that she was still bleeding vaginally and still having periods, examined her. Now he thought he had a somewhat more feasible explanation for her problem. He said it was possible that a section of placenta had been stitched into the womb and that a 'D and C', Dilation and Curettage, where the wombs lining is examined under the microscope, should be conducted and this material would be 'scraped' away. Chris's admission to hospital was arranged for Wednesday, 1 February.

She returned home with this news, emphasizing that it was a 'normal procedure' and that she would be in hospital only for the day. At last! There was now something positive happening. The consultant gynaecologist had finally diagnosed her condition. It seemed a satisfactory explanation and one that Chris could readily accept.

Chris was convinced this time that her long and painful ordeal was at last coming to an end. It never even entered our heads that a doctor's expert opinion could be so terribly wrong.

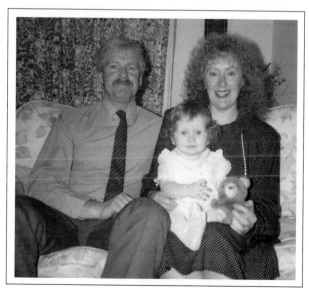

The day before Chris went into hospital

SEVEN

Your wife has cancer and she's going to die

Chris was admitted to hospital as planned on 1 February, 1989. A House Officer, a junior doctor, recorded a general examination and medical history. At the end of his notes he wrote: *For EUA and cx (cervix) biopsy*, meaning that Chris would undergo an examination of the uterus under anaesthetic and a sample of tissue from the cervix would be removed for diagnosis. The operation was to be performed the following day.

That evening, Chris appeared relaxed and optimistic as she sat up in bed, talking to the other patients. It seemed that all her worries were nearly over. At last a relatively simple operation would provide the key to her long-suffering condition. Three days earlier, she had been weighed at nine stone seven pounds; she seemed to be in reasonably good health. When I left, I was looking forward to her coming home the next day.

On the morning of Thursday, 2 February, I was working in my office at the dairy company, expecting a telephone call from Chris telling me that I could return to collect her. Rebecca was with her childminder. At eleven o'clock the phone did ring but it wasn't the call I had been waiting for. It was the ward sister, Hilary Frood. She asked me to come to the hospital straight away to talk with Group Captain Baxendall, concerning Mrs Lucey. She couldn't say any more.

I replaced the receiver, wondering why there was such an urgency to see Dr Baxendall. Perhaps Chris had to stay in longer or maybe he wanted to explain how pleased they were to have stopped the bleeding. All sorts of possibilities ran through my mind as I left for the hospital.

I was ushered into Dr Baxendall's office and asked to sit and wait. The ward sister closed the door behind me. Immediately I stood and began pacing up and down, my hands cradled together behind my back. At last the door opened and I rushed back to my seat, pretending that I had been sitting there patiently for the past few minutes. Dr Baxendall walked in. I stood up as he closed the door behind him. He said, "Sit down please," in his authoritarian voice. I sat, reacting like a puppy dog, obeying his master's command.

He approached me and placed his right hand on my shoulder. I did not have the time to ask how Chris was or to mention the operation. He offered no consultation, nor did he attempt to build up gently to the news that was about to follow. Instead, he simply said, "There's no easy way to tell you this: your wife has cancer and she's going to die."

I remained sitting, paralysed, for a few seconds. Dr Baxendall's shattering words resounded in my head; my whole body went numb. Then I stood up, shaking, the palms of my hands sweating profusely. I had a sudden urge to wash them. I looked across the office and saw a washbasin near to a window. The window looked onto the ward, conveniently situated for staff to observe patients while they completed their reports during the quiet hours of the night. I walked towards the basin, asking his permission in the process; he didn't answer. My hands were trembling as I pushed the nozzle of the antiseptic soap dispenser and began vigorously washing my hands. Dr Baxendall handed me a paper towel.

I could see through the partially opened venetian blinds into the ward. Most of the beds were occupied. I saw Chris midway down the ward. She was sitting up in bed reading; she looked perfectly normal. There were no signs of upset and I wondered if she knew. Had Dr Baxendall told her? I asked him and he said she had been told.

Desperately fighting back the waves of emotion I did everything I could to clear my mind and to regain some measure of control. Now, more than at any other time in my life, I needed to be strong.

But I found that I could not comprehend what was going to happen next. I knew nothing about cancer. I knew nothing of the many forms it took, nothing about its treatment. I did not even know what type of carcinoma Chris had or at what stage it was. She would know, of course, and from where I was standing she didn't look unduly worried. Perhaps, I kept telling myself, perhaps it wasn't all that bad. Doctors do make mistakes. If it was true that she was going to die, then why did she look so relaxed? I was utterly confused.

Dr Baxendall's voice interrupted these desperate thoughts. "Come on, I'll take you in to see her." As we walked onto the ward, Chris looked up. Normally, she would smile on seeing me, but not this time. She put her book down as I sat on the bed. Dr Baxendall gave a small cough and left us alone. A nurse, sensing our need for privacy, pulled partitioning curtains around the bed. Chris placed her arms around my shoulders; she seemed unmoved by the news. It was me that broke down. Holding onto her tightly I wept, "Cancer, Chris. He said you have cancer." I didn't repeat what he had said about her dying.

Chris hugged me and began reassuring me by saying that the cancer was probably in the early stages and with immediate treatment there was a good chance they could stop it from spreading. Obviously the news had been broken to her somewhat differently, not with the doom and gloom that accompanied Dr Baxendall's tactless approach to me. I began to hope against hope that perhaps it was not all that serious after all and told her that, if necessary, we would sell our house, She would have the best treatment possible, even if it meant going to America to receive it. She said that there was no better place than England to have the treatment and everything would be fine.

The biopsy of the cervix had revealed a poorly differentiated malignant tumour. Arrangements had been made to transfer Chris straight away to the Churchill Cancer Treatment Hospital in Oxford as an emergency case. There she would begin a course of radiotherapy and chemotherapy. She was to be conveyed by ambulance. I would follow in my car.

That hour-long, thirty-two mile journey was the longest and loneliest journey of my life. As I drove behind the old military-style ambulance, my thoughts ran over past events, recalling the numerous times Chris had said, "Thank God, Don. It's not cancer." Her worst fears had now become our reality. I thought how I would break the news to our families and friends. And, of course, I thought about Rebecca. She was only a year old but I knew how much she would miss her Mummy. So many issues swirled around in my head. Mile after long mile, I stared at the back of the ambulance, feeling distraught and helpless. Only a few days earlier we had been celebrating Rebecca's first birthday. We had been so happy. What cruel twist of fate could do this to us. Why did Chris deserve this?

Neither of us could know that this was only the beginning of a very long spell of hospitalisation that would continue for the next fourteen months. This journey would be the first of many for me. Our lives were about to change dramatically.

Chris was taken to the radiotherapy outpatient department and admitted for urgent assessment in preparation for a regimen of treatment to destroy the cancer cells. I left to go home to tell our family and friends but I had one place to go first. To save myself from going crazy, I had to shout at someone. I had to shout at God. I had to give Him a piece of my mind.

I parked my car outside the gate leading into Clouts Wood, in the village of Wroughton and walked down a track for a short while, away from people and habitation. I stopped and looked up into the dull clouds and screamed at the top of my voice, "Why us, God? Why? I don't believe in you any more. You're taking away someone I love. If You really did exist, You wouldn't take Chris from me."

It started to rain as I walked back to my car. I felt so bitter, the outburst had released the depths of my anger. Yet somehow I believed that God had heard me and that the rain was His way of saying how sorry He was and that He would do everything He could to help Chris recover. It made me feel better. It would help me to cope.

I went home and began the daunting task of telephoning everyone to tell them the news. I telephoned my mother first. My sister, Tina, answered and I asked to speak to Mum. When she came on the phone I found it difficult to talk, my vocal cords were locked. The shock of actually telling her that Chris had been transferred to Oxford for cancer treatment rendered me speechless. I tried in vain to say *something* but couldn't. The experience brought the memories flooding back of the time when I found my father. My speech had been incoherent then. This time it was worse. Mum sensed my distress immediately and just said, "It's all right, son, take your time".

Silence from me.

Then, "I love you. Take your time."

Tears rolled down my face as I began to stammer the news that Chris had cancer and was going to die. After a few minutes, I was finally able to converse in a more composed manner. My mother was wonderful. She offered her help and support and her understanding and kindness was to play an important role in the years that followed.

Next I informed Christine's parents. They made arrangements to come to our home. I received a somewhat different response from Chris's younger sister. To my utter amazement, she began shouting at me. "What do you mean she has cancer?" she screamed. "How can she possibly be going to die?" It was only her shock and disbelief causing her to vent her anger at someone, I was straight in the line of fire. But I could not help it. I was left with a feeling that I *was* somehow to blame.

I returned to see Chris later that evening. She had already started the treatment and had received a specified dose of radiotherapy. A small purple spot had been imprinted on the lower region of Chris's abdomen: this was a measurement mark to guide the radiotherapy beam; she was told it would be permanent. She had also had a blood transfusion. She looked miserable and was missing Rebecca.

My first impression of the Churchill Hospital was disappointing. A network of gloomy and eerie corridors led onto wards and medical departments, interlinking the post-war construction of Nissen huts. Chris was in Ward Seven, a mixed ward for patients with a variety of cancer-related illnesses. At the time of her admission it seemed an inappropriate ward for her. She looked so healthy and out of place in these depressing surroundings, filled with terminally ill patients, young and old, all suffering and in pain.

The nurses didn't wear uniforms. They were dressed in casual clothes; their name badges were marked informally, with scrolled Christian names and designed with pictures of smiley faces, teddy bears or sunflowers. They seemed to signify the characters and personalities of the individuals. Macmillan nurses, specially trained to care for cancer victims, were assisting on the wards.

Weary patients shuffled from bed to bed pushing along apparatus that contained catheters and their own individual infusion units of anti-cancer drugs. I saw them vomiting into bowls, their dignity long surrendered in the desperate quest for at least a temporary cure. The sight of these poor people left me feeling uncomfortable and depressed.

The hospital, named after Winston Churchill had been a military hospital for American servicemen during World War Two. Over the years additional buildings had been added, including a department that specialised in tropical diseases. Annually, it treated twenty-two thousand inpatients and fifty-eight thousand outpatients. Surgeons there performed ten thousand operations a year.

For the next two weeks, my daily routine was fixed. I went to work, travelled to Oxford to visit Chris and collected Rebecca from her childminder. Somehow I was able to find enough spare time to continue my regular running sessions, managing to maintain a reasonable level of fitness. I also found that the exercise helped me to release a lot of the tension that built up daily. It helped me cope with the stress.

Suddenly I had been thrown into the role of a single parent. It took a while for me to adapt to the mundane tasks of household chores and the more important role of caring for Rebecca. Our daughter began to take her first steps and I captured this important event on video to show Chris. I was determined to do everything I could so that she would not miss the real thrill of seeing her daughter walk and hearing the excitement in her tiny voice.

Chris was shortly to have a two-week break at home to recover from the effects of the treatment before returning for further therapy and she was discharged from hospital late in the evening of 18 February. She looked pale and ill, the treatment having taken its toll. Worse still, her homecoming lasted only a single day. She had to be readmitted to Princess Alexandra's Hospital, Wroughton, the following morning with severe vomiting and diarrhoea, an appalling, but common, adverse reaction to the treatment. Typically, Rebecca refused to demonstrate her newfound walking skills during the brief time that Mum was home.

After the fourteen-day course of radiotherapy at Oxford, Chris commenced chemotherapy on 13 February, the day after her thirty-fourth birthday. The anti-cancer drugs were administered through an intravenous and a central venous line. A special dye test had showed no evidence that the cancer had spread into the lymph nodes or that it had metastasised, spread to other areas of the body distant from the original tumour. Her chest X-ray revealed no evidence of lesions in her lungs and the X-ray of her urinary system proved normal.

However, there was an impression of a filling defect on the left side of her bladder, and an ultrasound of the pelvis revealed a large mass just behind the bladder. A CT scan of the abdomen and pelvis showed a soft tissue mass expanding from the cervix, which appeared to extend upwards into the uterus. This tumour was substantial.

EIGHT

Poisoned chalice

Chris had begun the first nightmarish course of chemical and radiation treatment: the horror of surgery was yet to follow. These combined treatments would eventually obliterate her body. Moreover, she was still oblivious to the real prognosis that was to come. Chris was never aware of the interpretative errors on her smear tests between 1977 and 1988, including the smear reported on 21 June 1988, *seven and a half months before* the diagnostic biopsy that discovered her cancer.

On 20 February, 1989, Chris returned to that same hospital ward where she had originally been given the dreadful news of her illness. Ward One was located on the first floor of the two-storey building and was, ironically, directly opposite the maternity unit where Rebecca had been born. An ante/postnatal and gynaecology clinic were situated midway along the corridor, with other rooms on either side that contained an Intensive Care Unit, staff rest room, kitchen, laundry and a patients' bathroom. A side ward was positioned near the main office and double-hinged swing doors led into the gynaecology ward.

The ward was divided into three sections that accommodated twenty-one metal-framed beds; each draped in a blue bedspread with white pillows. Each bed space was identically furnished with a small chair, wooden bedside locker and cabinet, wall-mounted electrical-audio control panel and an extending light fixture. French doors on the west side of the ward opened onto a long balcony that overlooked verdant lawns, flowerbeds and the main car park at the front of the hospital. Nearby were several two-storey buildings that accommodated servicemen and women; this was where Chris had lived before moving into rented accommodation in the village, twelve years earlier.

A day room for patients at the far end of the ward was used as a dining area and television lounge. A south-facing bay window three metres high let plenty of light into the room, and provided a glorious view of mature oaks, weeping willows, tall conifers, blossoming apple trees and all the other delights of the immaculately landscaped gardens. The Ridgeway, three miles away, was outlined on the horizon.

Patients requiring optimum nursing care were located near the front of the ward and were regarded as priority. Those needing less medical attention were in beds near the middle or end. Chris occupied the first bed on the right near the main office, whose window I had looked through onto the ward when that bombshell was dropped on me two weeks earlier. Staff could watch Chris more closely from this observation point and could monitor her condition when they were not on ward duty. If she required urgent assistance at any time, she could press an emergency call button on a remote control unit.

Chris's condition had deteriorated since her discharge from Oxford and she continued to vomit violently every two or three hours. It seemed impossible to control the poisonous side effects of the anti-cancer drugs on her body. She also had several bouts of diarrhoea and was prescribed a mixture of antibiotics. She was unable to digest anything properly and regurgitated the small amounts of food she attempted to eat. Even sipping small mouthfuls of water became an impossible and intolerable feat for her. These terrible nauseous and feverish symptoms gripped and twisted her organs, impairing their normal function and she perspired profusely. Her dampened nightwear required regular changing. She had showered and bathed several times that first day when I came to visit.

It fell to Dr Baxendall, who was now aware of all her smear results, and his team of doctors and nurses to play their part in helping Chris to recover from the devastating side effects of the chemical and radiation treatments. She had been anticipating some form of bad reaction, but had not expected it to be quite this terrible. A patient medical chart which depicted the physiological condition of her body: showed that a number of basic functions were well below the normal levels. The medical staff provided what professional assistance they could to nurture her back to health and attempted to counterbalance her sickness. An intravenous infusion was commenced and she was given Cyclizine, a drug used to treat nausea, intramuscularly at six to eight hour intervals. Chris needed to be strong enough to return to Oxford for a second course of treatment.

Her condition had not improved by the second day. A member of staff contacted the Churchill Hospital Oncology Department for advice and was informed that the vomiting and diarrhoea should eventually 'settle'. Chris was given fluids orally, including small amounts of food and 10 mg of Lomotil, a drug that relaxes spasm in bowel muscles.

By 22 February she was feeling much better, her diarrhoea had stopped and the infusion was suspended. She was, however, still nauseous. It was impossible to predict how long it would take for her to recover fully from the treatments. On Saturday, 4 March, Chris was transferred back to Oxford: her two-week 'recovery break' was over.

The demanding journeys to Oxford and Wroughton began to dominate my life. Each day I confronted and accommodated every eventuality of upheaval and disruption caused by Chris's unexpectedly prolonged stay in hospital. Chris's role as a mother was slowly declining: my wife and daughter were apart, separated from the normality of the everyday love they had once shared. Our household was turned upside down, each of us adapting and becoming dependent on each other for help and support. Chris's hospitalisation had eclipsed everything: including my career, social activities and free time.

Her parents arrived at our home on 8 February. Originally they had planned to visit and to spend time with their daughter on the eighteenth, until she returned to Oxford for the second stage of treatment. But Chris's mother became increasingly concerned about her condition and she decided to stay an additional four weeks. Her father, understandably, had to return home earlier because of work commitments.

Rebecca, with her early morning baby chatter, became my alarm clock. Her room was across the landing, opposite our main bedroom, and both doors were purposely left open as reassurance for me during the night. She slept in a wooden cot with adjustable safety railings on each side. Everything was in place, just as Chris had left it on Rebecca's first birthday. Her bedroom was decorated with Mr Men wallpaper, and a frieze of numbers and letters of the alphabet encircled the top and middle of the wall. Cardboard-cut-out circus animals and clowns dangled from the ceiling; 'My Little Pony' curtains framed the windows. Assorted toys were spread around the room or neatly stacked on shelves and other furniture.

Rebecca would awaken most mornings and stand, holding onto the panel at the end of the cot, excitedly bouncing up and down. Usually she would look towards my room, calling out for Chris or me in her baby gargle or she would sit chatting quietly to herself, playing with soft toys. This brief contentment allowed me time to shower and get dressed, before tackling the first task of changing her disposable nappy, and then bathing and dressing her. After breakfast I would take her in my car to the childminder's, and then my working day began.

My employers were compassionate and supportive. They allowed me to change my regular nine-to-five hours to facilitate the upheaval in my circumstances. I began to work flexible shifts each week, three hours one day, and usually four or five the next. My managerial position allowed me to delegate and share various responsibilities with departmental supervisors during my absence.

Every day I went to the hospital. I would drive along the main entrance road and stop at the military checkpoint near the officers' mess. Armed RAF policemen and soldiers stood guard near the sentry box and manually-operated barrier. There was always a flurry of activity as sentries checked everyone's identity passes. People arrived in private vehicles, while military transport brought personnel from other MOD establishments, including a military housing married quarters estate two miles away. Public transport operated a shuttle service to the isolated encampment, conveying civilian employees, day patients and visitors from local communities. Military helicopters flew regular sorties in and out of the grounds. Soldiers injured by urban terrorists on the streets of Belfast or from army manoeuvres on Salisbury Plain, were all brought here. Also, casualties evacuated and airlifted from overseas theatres of war were relayed from RAF Lyneham ten miles away, the same Air Force base where journalist, John McCarthy and church envoy, Terry Waite, arrived after being released as a hostage by Islamic Fundamentalists.

Ambulances full of paramedics and trauma teams frequently sped across the tarmac from the main entrance, ferrying victims of real and simulated war games from the designated helicopter-landing pad to the casualty department. Medical personnel, dressed in different coloured military uniforms of army, navy, and air force services, walked the labyrinth of footpaths leading from the junior ranks' accommodation to their places of work. Their hospital superiors: officers and senior ranks consisting of consultants, surgeons, anaesthetists, doctors and senior nursing staff, approached the same venue from the sergeants' quarters and officers' mess.

Each morning for two weeks, Chris's mother accompanied me to the hospital and stayed with her daughter for several hours. Occasionally I would take the opportunity either to return to work or to extend my running sessions along the Ridgeway. Some days I would run carrying a heavy Bergen rucksack on my back weighing sixty pounds or more. The weather could turn nasty in the blink of an eye out there in the countryside, especially during February, but I had always enjoyed the challenge of running in bad conditions and quickly acclimatised to freezing fog, snow, gale force storms or torrential rain. Often my sports clothes were drenched and I would have to change before returning to Chris.

During visiting time I would frequently discuss Chris's illness with Dr Baxendall or with the ward staff, but they would normally bewilder me with medical jargon relating to her intake of medication, lack of nutrition or the after-effects of her chemotherapy, which were only too obvious. Every time I left the hospital with her mother, she would break down and cry. Then we would collect Rebecca from her childminder and return home, until I visited again in the evening

NINE

Gloomy prospect

Having watched Chris endure these first four weeks in hospital, I found it hard to imagine how she was able to tolerate the constant medication and treatments and still have the will to continue. But as this medical tragedy unfolded I began to understand her psychological state more clearly.

Chris knew that her diagnosis was cervical cancer, presumably in the early stages, and believed that if it were treated quickly there was a good chance it could be prevented from spreading any further. The encouraging information she received from the medical fraternity helped to relieve some of her own doubts and fears.

Typically, she always wanted to know as much as possible about her disease; she consulted manuals and questioned the doctors. Chris was, after all, a trained nurse. She had a natural appetite to investigate the subject. She shared everything she discovered with me and I was inspired by her optimism, despite the trauma of watching her going through so much agony. Chris was very strong-minded: a born survivor.

Each day represented a new challenge for her, both physically and mentally. Her ability to endure such pain and suffering in this fight for survival was founded on the support I gave her, our commitment to each other and, of course, her love for Rebecca. At the beginning, our families and our friends were almost as important; though much later some of them were to lose faith in Chris's positive outlook.

Now Chris was about to start another course of chemotherapy and radiation therapy and to learn some very upsetting news on her prognosis. I stood by her bed next to her consultant oncologist, Dr Adrian Jones. We had regarded him as something of a saviour since he was said to be a radical oncologist and had the reputation of a 'Medical Boy Wonder'. At the onset of her therapy he had told Chris that he was hopeful but his optimistic attitude concerning her prognosis had changed.

He now told us that the prospect was gloomier than he had first thought. He was referring to the stage the disease had reached: not only had the cancer spread, but also it was the most aggressive that he had ever seen. Thus Chris's perception that her disease was in the early stages was shattered. Now she had nothing to hold on to. This was a severe blow to her morale. It seemed that all hope that the cancer could be stopped was now gone. She was terribly distressed.

I thought back to what Dr Baxendall had told me in his office. I had been mortified by his seemingly callous attitude and his negativity. But he had been right; he knew what he was talking about after all. Later, a member of staff on Ward Seven told us that Adrian Jones "was known to take risks in the management of radiotherapy and chemotherapy, especially where there was a chance that the risk would pay off." Right now we just wanted to know how much time Chris had left to live, but he would not commit himself to a time scale, simply telling us it was 'in the lap of the gods'.

Later that day, I had the opportunity to talk to him alone. I asked him about the treatment Chris had already received and the probability of success in future therapy, hoping against hope for some comforting words about her chances of survival. He told me there was no guarantee that the treatment would be successful; we would just have to wait and see. He also told me that she had a stage II malignant cancer. She would need all the support I could give her, her condition would worsen and ultimately it would affect our relationship. He explained the need to increase the dosage of both chemo and radiation therapies and warned me to expect even worse side effects than we had already witnessed. Chris would lose more weight and would experience total hair loss.

On 8 March, the fourth day of Chris's second course of treatment, she looked very unwell and felt extremely low. She was pining for Rebecca. Children were not allowed on the ward though occasionally Chris was able to leave the ward to see her.

I tried to cheer her up a little by saying that if everything went according to plan she might be allowed home for the Easter holidays and our family could all enjoy a few days together. She squeezed my hand in acknowledgement and said that she hoped so too. I still felt, however, that there was something else upsetting her and I asked what was wrong.

Chris began telling me about an article she had read in a magazine the previous day, that reported a link between cervical cancer and promiscuity. She had mentioned these details to a nurse and had said, obviously in confidence, that she hoped no one on the ward had thought she had been promiscuous. She had not dreamt that these comments would be repeated to anyone but, a little later, Dr Jones had made reference to the matter. Actually he berated Chris, saying he didn't care what sort of person she was, or what her sex life had been like, she was going to get the same therapeutic treatment as everyone else. This overreaction was clearly due to a misunderstanding of the communication she had had with the nurse. The breach of confidence had damaged her trust in the hospital staff. I told her not to worry too much about it. The other staff were probably much more discreet. Chris asked me not to confront Jones and the nurse about the incident, saying that she would deal with it in her own way. But I knew she would not forget their attitude and the lack of professionalism.

The incident did not affect my general admiration for all the staff in the hospital and in particular for the specially trained doctors and nurses on Ward Seven; their expertise and professionalism was a credit to the medical fraternity. Each day they were confronted with appalling human suffering, yet even as they observed the despair and trauma of their patients, they still managed an air of calm tranquillity and general cheerfulness.

Chris continued with the treatment regimen, and soon became too ill to care about this incident. She underwent some CT scans, a horizontal examination of the body able to detect the progression of groups of cancer cells.

On 23 March she was discharged from hospital and allowed home for the Easter holiday. It was to be a short break of only a few days, before returning for the last stage of treatment. She now weighed seven and a half stone, her hair was thinning and she was utterly exhausted. But thankfully it was nearing the end of this therapy, after which she would have a longer period at home to relax. Just three more days to go and that would be the end of the seemingly interminable bombardment of radiation and the endless cocktails of drugs. In fact, the sessions should already have been completed, but the radiotherapy had initially had to be suspended due to Chris's excessive sickness and diarrhoea during the middle of March.

The theory behind this two-stage, carefully calculated dosage of chemo and radiotherapy was that it could stop the cancer from spreading, thus preventing the need for surgery. It might even be sufficient to destroy the cancer completely. Closely monitored CT scans of the pelvic area would indicate any further signs of tumour growth and any future radiation treatment would depend on what showed on these scans.

There was also the final option of a hysterectomy, which would surgically remove the tumour and remaining malignant cells in the area. It all remained to be seen.

That Easter, Chris was so excited at seeing her baby again for the first time in ages. It was the moment she had been longing for over the past seven weeks. But her thin, drawn face could barely support a smile and, as she approached Rebecca, she broke down and began to cry. She held her tightly in her arms and started talking to her, saying that she only had three more days to stay in hospital and then she would be home for good. She hugged her as though she would never be able to let go and said she loved her very much and had missed her and Daddy. She never wanted to go back to hospital again because she was going to get better and we were all going to have a lovely Easter together. Then she pulled an Easter egg out of a bag and gave it to the daughter she'd missed so much.

Chris had made many friends in hospital, both among the nurses and the patients. One fellow patient was a young man called Stuart, whose twenty-first birthday was three weeks away. He had invited Chris and me to his party. He was having treatment for a brain tumour and had spent many months undergoing both extensive radiotherapy and chemotherapy. His shaven head also bore the scars of past surgery. Each day he had experienced intense bouts of loneliness and depression caused by mood changes relating to his illness and medication. This was the case with most patients on the ward. I had watched my own wife go through it.

When Chris had first entered Ward Seven, she did not seem to fit in with the other cancer patients, they all seemed so much more ill than she was. How rapidly that had changed.

Visiting was probably the most important part of the patients' day. Stuart would often ask Chris when I was visiting and he enjoyed chatting with me. Most of our conversation was about football, I did not support any particular team, but general football talk kept him happy. Chris had invited Stuart and his family to our home one weekend, and he often talked of meeting Rebecca. We had been told that he did not have long to live.

TEN

No other alternative

After our Easter break Chris returned to the hospital to complete the course of treatment. That particular stage of radiotherapy finished on Wednesday, 30 March, but no one could tell her how effective the large doses that she had received would be in the short term. It was now simply a case of waiting. She had remained optimistic throughout the treatment, even after she had learned how advanced her cancer actually was and her positive mental attitude had helped.

Chris continued to enquire about her life expectancy, but the vague response from medical staff only indicated that they could never be sure how effective their therapy had been. She began to feel like she had been taking part in an experiment, being used as the proverbial guinea pig. It seemed that their methods of administering the various drugs had always been based on trial and error principles.

When Chris was discharged from hospital on the 2 April, two further appointments were arranged: the first was for a CT scan at her local NHS hospital and this was to be followed by a return visit to Oxford on 17 April. At the second appointment she was to be examined under anaesthetic to consider whether she should have intra-cavity radiotherapy to complete her treatment. This would involve inserting wires or small tubes containing radioactive caesium into her uterus and leaving them there for a period of time. The alternative would be to offer a hysterectomy.

Over the course of two months, Chris received a 5000-cGy dosage of radiotherapy in two sets of treatment; the first given over a period of fifteen days, followed by a 'break' of fourteen days, which was initially intended for recovery at home, but spent in Princess Alexandra Hospital; the second over twenty-two days. An eight-day intermission in the second set was necessitated by the gravity of the side effects. Chris became feverish during this time and received additional medication involving four different types of antibiotics.

On 11 April she had another CT scan, her first at Princess Margaret's Hospital in Swindon. The anatomical horizontal scanner there was the only one in Wiltshire, an addition to the hospital equipment made possible through a long and arduous sponsored appeal by a local man, Richard Webb. This benefactor was a police officer and also a cancer victim who died from a brain tumour before the final total of a million pounds had been raised. The scanner was named in his honour and a memorial plaque is located in the Town Gardens in remembrance of his courage and commitment to society.

Every month Dr Jones would hold an oncology clinic at Princess Margaret's Hospital where patients could consult him regarding their individual therapy programmes. This helped to ease the congestion and backlog at his own clinic in Oxford and made appointments easier for outpatients who lived in the locality of Swindon and who would otherwise have been forced to travel sixty miles to his Oxford clinic. The option of waiting for his monthly Swindon clinic or travelling to see him at the Churchill Hospital in Oxford really depended on the seriousness of an individual's cancer. For many it was an essential pilgrimage to Oxford to continue with further radiation and chemical treatment. The results of Chris's scan would be made known to us on her re-admission to hospital on 17 April.

Amazingly, at this point she appeared to be in moderately good health. After eleven days at home, she was starting to gain weight again and had suffered no major setbacks this time as a result of the toxic treatments. She even began to enjoy the occasional day out. Unfortunately she was unable to attend our friend Stuart's birthday party and I went on my own.

When she was re-admitted on 17 April, the results of the CT scan showed there were no signs of any additional growth of the tumour. However, only the para-aortic region of the abdomen had been scanned; not the pelvis. The next day Chris was examined under anaesthesia. This determined the bladder to be normal, but the cervix was irregular. Small sections of Chris's cervix were pulled away with forceps and examined. The cervix was very fragile, and it was not possible to insert the radioactive caesium implant due to perforation of the uterus. An antiseptic pack was inserted for twenty-four hours.

Following these examinations, Dr Jones told Chris that the insertion of radioactive caesium could not be done because the tumour growth inside her cervix was too large, and that no more radiation therapy was possible. The following day we were told officially that she would have a hysterectomy on 1 May and that there was no other alternative. Chris was transferred to Princess Alexandra's Hospital the next day.

A telephone conversation on 21 April between Dr Jones and the newly promoted Air Commodore Baxendall confirmed the results of Dr Jones's examination, which stated that the cervix appeared friable but there was no evidence of spread outside the cervix. Neither did the CT scan show any evidence of spread. He also said that he had been unable to locate the cervical canal and therefore could not insert the radio-caesium. He now recommended a hysterectomy but advised that the lymph glands in the pelvic wall should not be included because this would cause severe lymphœdema or inflammatory swelling. Subsequently, we learned that this was a poor clinical decision. Lymphœdema is not a life-threatening condition. Whereas the tumour-involved lymph nodes, that identify spread, had occurred outside the uterus and needed to be removed.

I clearly recall the distress that the need for a hysterectomy caused Chris. She now had to come to terms with the fact that she would never be able to have any more children and it made her feel guilty because she thought she had let me down. She had hoped Rebecca would have a brother or sister one day, but now her world was in turmoil again, She had to face up to the fact that it was a choice between having this major operation or letting the cancer spread. This was not an alternative. It was hard for me to understand, at this stage of her illness, that her inability to conceive ever again concerned her so deeply

Dr Baxendall was very much aware of Chris's state of health externally and was soon to learn at first-hand the real status of her diseased body internally. With hindsight, we often wondered if he felt somewhat responsible for her illness. Perhaps his failure to recognise the early symptoms had translated into a guilt complex. At this point it seemed to us as though he was trying to make amends by ensuring she received the very best care possible. Chris was under the impression that she was rather an important patient and she assumed that her first-class treatment from Dr Baxendall and his medical team was simply because of her military background, plus the fact that she had once been stationed at the hospital as a nurse.

It so happened that, prior to Dr Baxendall starting his annual leave, he organised Chris's forthcoming operation personally, cancelled all leave for his team of medical staff and ordered the operating theatre to be opened on Bank Holiday Monday, May 1, 1989. This date would have a poignant significance six years later.

Chris spent a few days at home before being re-admitted on 27 April to prepare for the hysterectomy. During this time, I was responsible for her nursing care. She was still suffering from profuse sickness and diarrhoea and complained of moderate abdominal pains. Her medication consisted of a morphine elixir, for substantial pain relief; Ranitidine, to reduce acid secretion in the stomach; Stemetil, to relieve nausea and vomiting and codeine, for moderate pain relief. These various drugs were administered throughout the day and I made daily journeys to the local pharmacist to collect the prescriptions.

On Thursday, 27 April, Chris was admitted to Princess Alexandra Hospital for a laparotomy; this would involve making a surgical incision through the abdominal wall to allow investigation of abdominal organs. However, Chris was clearly in no fit condition to have a laparotomy. Medical staff noted that she was exhausted, weak and lethargic, and complained of intermittent pain on the left side of her pelvis. She was also nauseous, vomiting and anorexic, and had an offensive vaginal discharge. A blood count showed that her haemoglobin level was low.

On April 28, Chris was feverish, constipated and taking very little food by mouth. She had vomited twice during the previous night. She was given a phosphate enema that produced improved bowel movement and she received two units of blood overnight. The following day she was feeling much better and began to tolerate oral fluids and food. A further enema was arranged. On 30 April it was recorded that she had diarrhoea three times the night before, possibly caused by Picolax, a laxative she had been given. But her bowel clearance was said to have been very successful and she was feeling much better.

Dr Baxendall was at last able to perform the laparotomy as well as the hysterectomy on the first of May. Chris spent twelve hours in the operating theatre, receiving two units of blood, followed by a further two units administered post-operatively.

Later that day Chris was informed of his findings. Dr Baxendall said that the operation was not completely successful because he was unable to remove the entire tumour as it was stuck to other organs. He had removed what he could. He told Chris that he hoped that the piece of tumour he had not removed was now dead, as a result of the onslaught of radio and chemotherapy. She was also told that some of her womb had been removed. When I spoke to Chris later, she said that he had sounded optimistic.

I was only to find out very much later that this partial hysterectomy had been anything but successful .The cervix, which was the seat of the tumour had not been removed. Nor had the lymph glands, which can carry cancerous cells away to other parts of the body. There was, in fact, no malignant material in any of the tissue that *had* been removed. A very radical operation was in fact required and additional expertise should have been requested in order to perform it.

On 2 May Chris was slowly recovering. Her drains and vaginal pack were removed. The nurses on the ward tried to get her to walk to the washroom and dining room, but she was far too weak and fell over when she got out of bed. It was really only now that Chris realised she might die as a result of her illness. This hit me forcibly too; mostly because it was the first time I had seen such a change in her positive attitude. She looked terribly ill and so close to death. I think that her prime concern at this point was how much time she had left. The will to go on fighting seemed to have fled her weak and exhausted body.

She was so sure she could not survive much longer that she began asking the doctors and nurses how long she had to live. Of course, they didn't know. At one point she told me she believed in life after death and asked me if we could agree a password we could use to communicate after she had gone. We agreed on 'happy-go-lucky', because of my easy-going nature. She told me that if I used these words after she died, she would know that I was trying to contact her.

Yet I managed to convince myself that somehow she would pull through and I left her that evening holding onto my own belief that she would be fine. And, miraculously, over the following three days she began slowly to recover.

On 5 May, Chris was feeling a lot happier and her normal, confident attitude was coming back. I was in a side ward with our friend, Julie, taking comfort in Chris's partial recovery when an unwelcome visitor arrived.

I had come to learn that whenever Sally Black, Dr Jones's oncology nurse, walked into the room she was rarely the bearer of good news. In fact, I would later nickname her 'The Prophet of Doom'. Today, hers was a most untimely and unannounced visit, but fortunately Chris had already been informed of her random tactics and was expecting her to arrive one day. Sally Black was renowned for her blunt forecasts on the life expectancy of oncology patients. These did not apply only to 'terminally ill' hospice patients; she also dispensed her 'wisdom' to those who were not so branded – yet.

I remember her visiting patients on the cancer ward in Oxford and saw how they reacted as she explained their prognosis. They were already distressed and it was terribly upsetting for their families and everyone else to observe them becoming even more dejected. Chris gave comfort where she could whenever fellow patients confided in her or wanted to share their fears and she was persistent in encouraging them to fight on and not give up. But Nurse Black seemed unable to afford anyone the support they were seeking.

None of the staff knew that this woman was arriving that afternoon to see Chris, which, to my mind, called into question Sally Black's ethics. This unannounced visit was about to have severe repercussions, resulting in her abrupt exit from the hospital.

She began by asking Julie and me to leave the room, as she wanted to have a private and extremely confidential conversation with Chris. She said that Chris could discuss it with us later if she wished. Her talk would not take long, as she was extremely busy. Chris introduced me as her husband and said that she could say whatever she had come to discuss in front of all of us. Nurse Black sat near Chris and held her hand. She said she had been sent by Dr Jones to tell her that there was nothing more that could be done medically. Despite the surgery, the cancer was so aggressive that it would kill her very soon and she must face up to the fact she was going to die. Sally Black was there to help her to accept this she told Chris that she must prepare herself mentally. She must also ensure that her relatives and friends were fully aware of the seriousness of her disease.

The abrupt announcement of this 'death sentence' and the woman's tone of voice startled and alarmed Chris. She became agitated; tears filled her eyes. When she started to cry, she told the nurse to get out of the room, she said that she had no right to be the bearer of such news. The ward sister heard the commotion and came into the room, asking what had happened. Chris explained that she did not need anyone to tell her that she was going to die; she already knew how serious her illness was.

The ward sister left the room and returned a few minutes later with Dr Baxendall. He told the oncology nurse to leave the hospital immediately and not to return. He apologised to Chris and said he would speak with Dr Jones about the incident. Once again Chris had had to withstand an unnecessary episode of humiliation. A few days earlier she had been close to death and was still in the process of trying to recover. This was the last thing she wanted to hear.

I was soon to discover that this untimely conversation somehow gave Chris the determination to live.

ELEVEN

I'd rather die than have a stoma

A strange and unsettling period followed, full of distraught and unpredictable moments, but by 10 May, Chris was much more content. She seemed happier and was beginning to feel that she would soon be strong enough to come home for the weekend.

On 11 May she appeared to be improving, but just before nine that morning she began to feel nauseous and started vomiting again. A junior doctor carried out an abdominal and rectal examination and felt what appeared to be a large mass of tissue in her pelvic area, approximately the size of a twenty-week pregnancy. The initial thought was that it was a haematoma, a build-up of clotting blood, though there were no indications of low blood flow. Normal eating and drinking was stopped and intravenous fluids were administered. The following day Chris remained unwell and an ultrasound indicated that the mass was indeed a large haematoma. Later that day, a histology report showed there was no visible evidence of malignancy in small samples taken from the tissue mass.

Chris continued to suffer with abdominal pains, vomiting and nausea for the rest of the day. At 10:20 pm, when a senior consultant examined her, she had a high temperature and her pulse had also risen. He decided that the haematoma required draining and at 11:30 she was taken to theatre, where the original scar was opened and a large foul-smelling intra-abdominal abscess containing pale brown fluid was identified. The abscess cavity was about five inches deep and it was impossible to define any anatomy. There was, in fact, no active bleeding and no blood clot. It was decided that, in view of the findings from the previous operation on 1 May, no attempt would be made to define the abdominal structures, probably because of the tumour, being fused to various organs, it made identification impossible. A large bore tube was inserted to allow the abscess to drain and Chris began another course of antibiotics, which were administered intravenously.

On 13 May she began to feel more comfortable, her temperature was near normal and there was little drainage from the wound. Drip-feeding was recommenced.

But the day after this, another problem caused her further distress and anxiety. A feculent discharge had started seeping out of the wound. This was the first sign that Chris had a faecal fistula, which is a communication channel from the bowel to the outside of the body. Later that day it became more severe; the discharge more copious. It was decided that she would need a colostomy or 'stoma', which is a drainage from the bowel onto an external surface. Chris was assured that it was only a temporary measure and that it should be reversed after about six weeks.

Naturally, she was again terribly upset. I enfolded her in my arms as I had done a hundred times before. I had never even heard of the words, 'stoma' or 'colostomy', let alone understand the physical changes that this procedure would effect. Chris did. She told me she would rather die than have a stoma. It was the final straw; she had been through enough. Yet she knew there was really no alternative.

Chris had known elderly patients who had urostomy and colostomy pouches and she understood how they functioned. Her real concern was not just about being disfigured or feeling degraded, it was the physiological barrier it would create between us.

She was a young woman and still cared about her body image. She had tolerated her desecrated internal organs being dissected. The cancer was being destroyed by these procedures. She had coped with the humiliation of embarrassing sickness and major surgery, but now this was an even bigger psychological blow to her diminishing morale and self-esteem. Her physical appearance had changed yet again after the hysterectomy but so far she had escaped conspicuous external mutilation.

I was consoling Chris when the ward sister came into the side room carrying a silver tray and small decanter of sherry with three glasses. Hilary poured out three small glasses of sherry and said she thought that we all deserved a drink, for purely medicinal purposes, of course. It was a lovely gesture and certainly helped us to absorb the shock of yet another traumatic occurrence. The sister told Chris not to worry; it was only a provisional step to allow time for the ruptured bowel to heal. Chris was somewhat reassured and agreed to have the operation.

After it was performed on 14 May, Chris was transferred to Ward Ten, a surgical ward. For the following three days she was taken back to the operating theatre each day to have her dressings changed. Her temporary colostomy was active and performing with no complications.

On 17 May her haemoglobin had dropped substantially and a three-unit blood transfusion was arranged. Since there was difficulty in locating a vein in her arm, the intravenous infusion was sited in her left foot. The drain from the abscess was removed on the next day. The wound was very clean and healing well.

On 19 May Chris complained of excruciating pain in her abdomen, spreading through to her back, and she was given vast amounts of pain relief during that day, though no obvious cause for the pain was diagnosed.

Every new day brought some form of affliction. Chris's morale was low but she retained her will to recover. It was now 23 May and the next problem to arise was a faecal fistula of the pelvic wound itself. This meant that Chris now had to stop eating solid food again and was fed by drip. The anaesthetist reinserted a central venous line in the vein beneath the collarbone. This continued for two days. She also had a urinary catheter fitted but it was removed when it caused symptoms of urinary tract infection. The faecal discharge continued and caused contamination of the pelvic wound.

On 30 May it was decided that she should be taken to the operating theatre for another examination under anaesthesia and a washout enema. Later that day she returned to have a pelvic wound washout, again under general anaesthesia, which also included cleaning the colostomy. Once cleaned, the pelvic wound could be seen to be granulating. This meant that healing tissues were forming. Both the wound and the colostomy looked healthy. The effluent was clear but the fluids did not flow into the pelvis or rectum. The surgeon wrote on the operative records that this suggested there was a rectal fistula.

It was to take a further ten days before Chris was well enough to be allowed home for the weekend. It was now 10 June. When we arrived home, I opened the passenger door to help Chris out of the car. I remember how she raised both legs wearily, as though they were anchored to the foot well and then eased herself slowly around on the seat, placing her feet on the driveway. The pink mule slippers and her blue and green tracksuit looked enormous on her withered frame, like someone who was a size ten wearing a size sixteen outfit. She had lost over four stone in eighteen weeks and now weighed five stone.

Chris struggled to find the energy to raise the rest of her fragile torso out of the car and reluctantly used my arm for support as she levered herself upright. It was typical of her tenacity, still trying to be independent no matter how ill she was. She would not have it any other way.

She managed a smile, said it was good to be home and when she saw the home-made sign that read WELCOME HOME, MUMMY draped in front of the garage door, she said, "Thank you, Don, what a lovely surprise." I told her that Rebecca had helped me to paint the large words on the old bed linen and that her daughter was very excited about her coming home. Chris was shuffling along the path towards the front door when Rebecca ran out, calling, "Mummy, Mummy," and they fell into each other's arms.

Rebecca clutched her mummy tightly as they walked slowly towards the house. Back in the comfort of her own home, Chris would hopefully begin to regain her strength. She looked reasonably well, despite her thin and ravaged body, but her faintly spoken words were slurred.

Lying on the settee, she watched in delight as Rebecca played happily in front of us. Our daughter's early faltering footsteps had now turned into something much more confident. She was already attempting to construct simple sentences. The hours passed quickly as we watched her curious antics and entertaining ways. That night Rebecca and Chris shared the same bed. I took the spare bedroom.

It was a decision that would set the precedent for the remainder of our relationship.

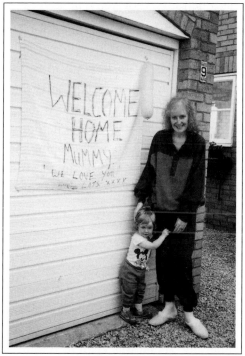

Welcome home, mummy

TWELVE

Complementary therapy

Chris returned to the hospital on Sunday evening and continued to receive close medical attention for the next three weeks. The pelvic wound was healing slowly. She was discharged on 4 July. An appointment was arranged for September, when it was intended she would have a barium enema to enable an investigation of her large bowel by X-ray, which would decide whether it would be possible to close the colostomy.

I was not happy that she had been discharged because she was still having horrendous bouts of nausea and vomiting. I carried a bowl as we walked slowly to the car and she vomited on the way home and complained of being in pain. It continued like this for the next six days. There was no actual decline in her condition but when the local doctor attended, his first priority was to send me to the pharmacist for an additional supply of morphine. Since he could see that Chris was in no fit state to be kept at home, he immediately contacted the hospital and had her re-admitted.

We were indeed fortunate to have our principal GP, Dr Peter Swinyard, living nearby. He was always helpful and considerate and gave Chris invaluable assistance in coping with her illness. As it happened, she was discharged again the following day, the symptoms of severe cramping in her upper abdomen and back pain had cleared after she had vomited profusely throughout the night.

*

Chris had collected some literature on complementary therapy and our GP thought she should give this a try. He felt that a different diet might help her to regain weight and could benefit her health generally. As he was keen to try anything that would give her the chance to fight the disease, she contacted the Bristol Cancer Help Centre. She arrived at Grove House in Bristol on Sunday 13 August for a week's residential course on complementary therapy and started 'The Bristol Programme' that same day.

There are many theories relating to the way cancer cells originate and develop, and some research seems to suggest that habit and diet contribute to their development. The theory behind the Bristol programme was a special daily diet of wholefoods such as whole grains and pulses which are believed to contribute to the body's physical, mental and spiritual health. The recommended foods both improve nourishment and help to eliminate toxins that build up in the body, allowing more efficient functioning of the organs. Chris had lost so much weight that she was given a specially modified diet: a typical daily menu consisted of:

Breakfast: Muesli with a little goat's milk, yoghurt and fresh pears and grapes.

Mid - morning: Fresh apple and orange juice.

Lunch: Raw salad of lettuce and chopped hazelnut with sprouts, beetroot leaves, chives, mint, wholemeal bread.

Mid-afternoon: Cup of rosehip tea, rice cakes with banana, and orange spread.

Dinner: Large portion of brown rice salad either hot or cold, grated beetroot and onion salad with chopped nuts, apple and wheatgerm surprise.

Before Bed: Cup of elderflower tea, with 1/2 teaspoon of honey, and a little lemon to taste or Slippery Elm drink.

A selection of other meals was available; including soups, casseroles and desserts. Anyone starting the diet would initially lose up to five or six pounds during the week- long course, mainly due to the lack of salt that enabled the body to eliminate fluids more quickly.

The centre also recommended a gradual change to the patient's usual eating habits prior to commencing the course. This was to avoid a shock to the digestive system and to assist in the alteration of daily routine and thinking processes. People generally had some entrenched eating patterns, usually going back to childhood and the transition to an entirely new diet could be difficult. It was also recommended that the partner or family should participate in the new dietary changes; this would support the patient in preparing the food and would avoid segregation of diets or the patient feeling different and lonely.

The Centre accommodated patients with most types of cancer and the therapy included helping them to adopt a positive attitude towards building a stronger and healthier body and mind. Relaxation was important and they encouraged Chris to seek the help of a spiritual healer, to practise yoga and to listen to soothing music. One of her favourite methods in this healing process was to stand in the shower and imagine that the flow of water was washing away all the infection from her body. This would rejuvenate her as she imagined the cancer being flushed down the drain.

NB: The nutritional guidelines and therapeutic content of the courses at the Bristol Cancer Help Centre do change from time--to-time; for up-to-date information see useful contacts, page 190.

When Chris returned from Bristol, I could see that the new dietary regimen and the adoption of a more positive mental attitude had benefited her considerably. I continued to participate in the preparation of her diet but I never became converted.

Chris continued to be supported by our family and friends and the general perception was that no one had to worry about me. After all, Chris was the one who had cancer and was going through so much pain and suffering. I still had my health. I just had to cope with my own stresses. I had my career and I maintained a high level of physical fitness. Regular long-distance running, pounding mile after mile on the bleak hills and valleys of the local ridgeway terrain, helped me release my stress and exasperation.

The only two people who ever thought of my mental well-being and offered me consolation were my mother and my close friend, Alan. Mum would always ask how I was coping and begged me to contact her if ever I needed to talk. Alan would often arrange to meet up with me in the local pub near the hospital. I was able to confide in him totally.

I had temporarily suspended my training with the Territorial Army and the spare time I had at weekends was used for hospital visits and looking after Rebecca and Chris when she was home on release from hospital as she was unable to manage any household chores. She would spend the majority of the time just resting, normally lying on the sofa in our lounge. She would receive and make countless telephone calls. So many people were anxious about her health.

By now I was becoming an expert in the role of carer, I could manage everything from nursing duties to household tasks. I was beginning to understand how difficult it must have been for my mother and for the millions of other women who have to cope daily with their children for many years, often with no help or relief.

In the end I just did everything without thinking; it became my duty. If Chris wanted medication, food or drink, it was there beside her. If friends or visitors arrived, I would entertain them. I became a self-taught master chef, preparing food for everyone, from midday snacks to three-course meals. I could accomplish all of the household chores with ease. No one seemed to care too much about all my additional duties; most of the time it was just expected. Except for the odd occasion when family members stayed, the majority of people who came to visit Chris just talked, rather than offering to help.

Chris had experienced dramatic changes both physically and mentally over the previous six months, her once attractive long blonde hair was now thinning and unsightly, her young body resembling that of a much older woman. The closeness that we shared helped us to withstand those early physical changes to Chris's body and our empathy for each other helped me to adjust to the way her body had become. When you share an absolute love, as ours was, when you have enjoyed so much of life together, nothing can break that bond. Supporting one's partner becomes almost second nature. Inevitably, I thought about our wedding vows: *to love, honour and obey, in sickness and in health, till death do us part.* I would not forget my pledge to Chris. I knew that if I'd been the one to become ill, she would have supported me too.

Chris now looked frail and ghastly; she wore a colostomy bag located on the surface of her abdomen. This carried faecal matter and required frequent emptying; it omitted a distinctive pungent odour, which mingled ineffectively with a neutralising deodoriser she used. The bathroom cabinet, normally reserved for feminine articles such as make-up and *eau de toilette*, now housed a mixture of sanitary towels, colostomy pouches and their associated accessories alongside my razor and aftershave lotion. Chris was always so grateful that none of these awful details had to be shared with anyone else, even close family and friends.

For us, it had become normal. It was but a foretaste of what was to come.

THIRTEEN

The Last Rites

On 25 August Chris returned to hospital for the planned barium enema and X-ray. This procedure would give doctors an insight into the condition of the pelvic area and would indicate any flaws associated with her colostomy. They were hoping it would be possible to reverse the colostomy but their findings showed that it was malfunctioning. It was decided that she should have a defunctioning procedure to alleviate bowel blockage and surgery was arranged for 5 September.

Before this operation took place, Chris had discussions with the two consultants ultimately responsible for the management of her radiotherapy and surgical treatment. She discovered that they both had bizarre answers to her questions about her present condition. There appeared to be some medical conflict between Drs Jones and Baxendall.

Dr Jones had informed Chris that the partial hysterectomy operation, performed because the planned total hysterectomy that had to be aborted because the tumour was stuck to other organs, had been done too soon after the radiotherapy treatment. Dr Baxendall's reaction to these comments was even more sinister, though it seemed to justify a pressing need for the surgery. He told Chris that the radiotherapy treatment had caused the bowels to weaken; and this was proven during the operation as the bowels were falling apart in his hands.

Their conflicting opinions made no difference at this stage. By now the damage had been done either way. Chris knew that if she were to survive, the best option would be to accept more surgery. She did not relish the thought of any further radiation treatment.

The complications continued: during the operation the surgeons discovered that the colostomy was 'recessed' below the surface of the skin, and faecal matter had passed from the middle to the end loops, rather than going directly into the colostomy bag. They excised the skin around the colostomy and made a bridge of skin underneath the loop to position the colostomy correctly on the outside of the abdomen.

Chris was discharged on September 20, her colostomy now working satisfactorily. She returned to the hospital for regular check-ups over the following two weeks, during which time she had noticed that she was passing urine through her vagina and she mentioned this to Dr Baxendall. An X-ray examination revealed that the flow of urine was indeed passing through the bladder and exiting through the vaginal cavity. Another distressing episode was about to begin.

She was admitted to hospital once again on 14 November and more tests followed. A procedure was then performed whereby X-rays were used to monitor the flow of urine. There was evidence of reflux, a backward flow of urine from bladder to kidney and the bladder capacity was somewhat reduced. Chris actually had a hole in her bladder. Ultrasounds performed at the same time showed the kidneys and liver to be normal, with no evidence of tumours.

On 16 November a CT scan was carried out, investigating an area from the top of the liver to the perineum, the skin between vagina and anus, and this showed an irregular soft tissue mass just in front of the sacrum. The radiologist suspected that most of this was due to radiotherapy damage and the only area where she suspected tumour recurrence was on the left side at the vault of the vagina, between the rectum and the upper margin of the bladder. No tumours were demonstrated in the liver.

It was decided that Chris would need an ileal conduit, a diversion of urine into an external bag and that she should return for a urostomy. Both these stomas would become permanent features. Chris asked if it was possible to have a total pelvic clearance and her request was granted.

She was readmitted for further surgery on 1 December. At that time she was unable to walk without becoming exhausted and she still could not look after Rebecca without help but she was gaining some weight and felt better than she had done for some time.

On Monday, 4 December, the day of the operation, I awoke at 3:30 am. I decided to go into work at 4:15 am prior to visiting Chris before she underwent surgery, which was scheduled for 8:30 am. We were told that it was going to be a long and dangerous procedure and probably the most difficult operation yet.

It was 5:20 am when I walked into the ward and sat on a chair next to Chris's bed. She was still asleep. Staff Nurse Kim Lovak brought me a cup of tea. I read the newspapers and waited for Chris to wake up. I had spent so much time in the hospital over the previous eleven months that I was allowed to ignore the normal visiting hours, especially before an operation. Chris was awake by 6:00 am, and I knew that she felt better because I was at her side. We spent an hour reassuring each other and I left as they prepared her for the operation.

The notes taken on her operation that day indicated that during the procedure Chris received five units of blood, followed by a further four units that were transfused after the operation. The operation lasted until 4:45 pm. She had been in theatre for eight and a quarter hours.

The operation had been successful but Chris would never remember anything about the events that were to follow over the next several days. She lay in the recovery unit for the rest of that night, oblivious to the world around her, while the medical team battled to stabilise her condition.

I returned home that evening and telephoned our immediate families to update them. Everyone contacted the hospital frequently to enquire about her general health, but they still expected me to keep them informed of daily progress.

Chris's condition remained unchanged during the night. On 5

December her pulse rate had risen to 160 instead of the normal 50 to 80 beats per minute. Her blood pressure was disturbingly low and falling: her central venous pressure was abnormally high and rising. She had peripheral oedema and a chest X-ray showed plethoric lungs, suggesting that she had been over- transfused. She appeared to have received approximately six and a half litres of fluids, with an output of only two and a half litres, presumably from intravenous infusions of fluids from the previous day. Her serum potassium was low and had to be boosted and her blood clotting function was abnormal.

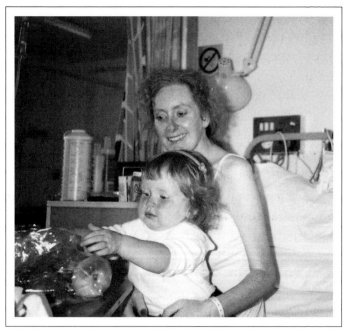

Chris and Rebecca, 1989

The surgical team reviewed her during the night and administered a diuretic intravenously to increase her urine output. Her condition worsened and on Wednesday, 6 December she was transferred to the Intensive Care Unit. It was now thought that she had septicaemia, blood poisoning.

Later that day the pelvic pack was removed and the doctor could see the small bowel through a defect in the wound. A small pack was inserted to close the opening and to protect the bowel. Five units of blood platelets were administered and by five o'clock her total protein had risen. A physiotherapist tried to help her loosen the sputum in her chest, as she was not able to cough very well.

On 7 December, she had a rapid respiratory and pulse rate. A further chest X-ray showed little change from the day before. More diuretic was given, as well as bicarbonate to correct her metabolic acidosis. At five o'clock that afternoon her potassium had dropped again and replacement was commenced.

By 6:30 pm she was reported to be in a very poor condition; more diuretic was given and a good passing of urine was obtained. There was cellular inflammation in her left flank that was spreading and a concentrated dose of penicillin was added to the antibiotics already being dispensed.

I was allowed to see Chris that evening. Her bed was considerably elevated and was surrounded by every conceivable piece of medical equipment associated with intensive care units. An oxygen mask covered her mouth and nose and numerous intravenous tubes trailed from her upper body. An array of medical charts lay on the floor nearby. Doctors and nurses stood around; each engaged in his or her individual task, still trying to stabilise her body from the trauma of surgery.

I sat in a small leather armchair near her bed, an odd and somewhat strange entity that seemed out of place amongst all the hospital furnishings and equipment. But it was probably an essential and temporary comfort used by ICU night staff as they sat and observed her condition while checking various monitors and drip pumps that pulsed a variety of fluids into her body.

Chris appeared lifeless, her head was tilted to one side and her eyes gazed downwards towards the floor, with me now in view. I was sitting considerably lower than her, my position awkward and uncomfortable. I reached out and held her hand. It felt cold and clammy. Her veins protruded above the surface of the skin and were an unusual grey-blue colour. Her thinning fair hair was darkened by beads of perspiration, and was brushed backwards.

I looked into her weary eyes, which she struggled to keep open. The oxygen mask covering her face seemed to emphasise the fatigue in those pale blue eyes gazing back at me. Her breathing was erratic and noisy and she was obviously in great pain; it seemed that her life was slowly fading away. Her eyes began to close. I could do nothing except clasp her hand and watch the activity of the medical staff around me, their non-verbal actions indicating that there really was no hope for her this time.

The ward sister beckoned me outside and asked me to seriously consider contacting Chris's relatives. She thought they should be nearby as she was in a critical condition. The doctors held little hope that she would last the night. The hospital padre was summoned and was waiting in the office when I went to use the phone there; he was prepared to perform the last rites.

I searched my mind, trying to find the right words to say to her parents as I picked up the receiver and dialled the number. The line was engaged. I replaced the receiver and walked out of the office. When I walked past the intensive care room the padre was standing near her bed with a bible in his hands. The sister came out and asked if Chris's family were on the way. I told her that I was unable to contact anyone as the line was busy. I said that I would try again when I arrived home. The sister urged me to keep trying on the office phone, but I said I wanted to do it in my own home. She walked off, obviously bewildered at my decision.

No one else had the authority to contact Chris's family, as I was her next of kin. It was up to me to make the decision. I knew that everyone wanted me to have her family present but I was now thinking differently. It was an odd position. I had the power to decide whether or not Chris should be allowed to die quietly, with only me present or to have everyone around her watching as she passed away.

As I trudged along the corridor leading to the hospital chapel, Chris's brother, Stephen, and his wife, Diane, were walking towards me. They were totally unaware of the present situation. I explained the circumstances and they both started to cry, accepting that this indeed was the end because the medical staff were of the same opinion. Stephen and Diane wanted to plead with the doctors to let Chris die soon. Their attitude was that she had suffered enough. I just said that she wasn't going to die, that she would pull through and that they should try to help her by being more optimistic.

They made their way to the staff rest room to smoke their cigarettes and seek sympathy from the hospital staff. I carried on my way to the chapel, carrying the bouquet of flowers they had brought for Chris. I knelt down near the altar and prayed to God to let my wife live for Rebecca's sake. They both needed each other. It wasn't fair to separate them.

After a while, I was conscious of the padre's presence again. He and a few other people were standing nearby, talking quietly to each other. Growing up as a Roman Catholic, I had always been cautious of small groups of people congregating around priests. I remembered how they always seemed to pause in conversation when someone drew near, hoping perhaps for a titbit of gossip, something to feed their rumour-mongering Then the talk would continue once the individual had passed, the poor unfortunate now almost certainly the sole topic of conversation.

I ignored the group's presence and kept repeating the Hail Mary over and over in my head. It was religious therapy, the Catholic method of scaring away evil and the impending spectre of death. Instinct told me that the padre was watching me, obviously concerned and waiting to express his condolences. I felt uncomfortable and agitated and discreetly looked behind; they were all staring in my direction. The padre bowed his head and then nodded sympathetically, his solemn expression and his look of compassion prompting me to end my prayers.

I exited on the opposite side of the chapel and thus avoided conversation. The last thing I wanted was an in-depth chat with the padre but I did not want to be overly rude. I gestured that I would speak with him later. I could not face anyone at that moment, certainly not someone who was negative to me. The padre would have reassured me that Chris would soon be at peace, and in the hands of God. Well, I did not want to hear any such thing. As far as I was concerned, Chris was not going anywhere. She was staying right here with Rebecca and me.

I placed the flowers on the altar and left for home. No, Chris was not ready to surrender to God just yet. Somehow, I was confident that she would have the strength to pull through.

I did not telephone her parents that night; my reasons were clear in my mind. I knew that if her family travelled down from Durham and Chris saw them gathered around her bedside, she too would lose her own belief in the possibility of survival and the determination to live.

It was a gamble I had to take. If she died, then I would have to face the fact that I had been wrong and had to accept the consequences.

FOURTEEN

I think she can do it

That night I was at home on my own. Rebecca was staying with her childminder. It probably seemed selfish of me not to have stayed with Chris but somehow I felt that my absence would inspire her to regain the will to live, so that she could see me again.

I telephoned the ward at eleven o'clock and was told that her condition was still deteriorating. I asked them to phone me if there was any change and went to bed at midnight.

Early the next morning the familiar buzzing of the telephone startled me out of what had been, strangely, a relatively good night's sleep. It was 6:40 am on Friday, 8 December. I awoke slightly disorientated, not quite sure who was calling at that time, but I soon recognised the voice. "Hello, Don, it's Kim from the hospital... " My heart began to pound; my senses slowly became aware of the reality of the previous night; a flashback of Chris lying in the intensive care unit. I sat up in bed as Kim continued: "Good news! Chris is awake and sitting up in bed, chatting away to everyone. She wanted a cup of tea, and is asking to see you. Her condition is much better, although it is still serious. It's great news, isn't it?"

I told her that I would come up straight away. Shortly after replacing the receiver, I telephoned Chris's parents and told them the news. My gamble had paid off. I had made the right decision. Now they could travel the three-hundred-mile journey to see her, if they wished. I explained that her condition had been critical overnight but I had decided that it was best not to worry them unduly, partly because of the distance and the lateness of the evening and also because of my theory about the negativity that would be generated by everyone gathering around Chris's bed.

They asked me to give her their love and said they would phone the hospital later that day to see how she was.

Nobody ever knew that I was not totally alone in making my decision that night. Something else had occurred that gave me a little encouragement but it was not a voice from God or a visit from an angel. Not only did I have my own belief that Chris would somehow pull through, but also someone else gave me a glimmer of hope when I needed it most, when everyone else had practically given up.

I happened to get into conversation with an ICU doctor, who said that I should go home that night and try to get some rest. He saw no point in my staying, because there was nothing I could do that would help. He said that no one could change the course of events that were to follow. If Chris was strong enough then she would survive. They would do everything to ensure she received the best medical assistance. When I asked him what he thought personally, he said, "I think she can do it." Hearing those six words helped me beyond measure.

However, when Chris learned later from the medical staff how she had come so close to death and of the decision I had made not to tell her parents, she made me promise that if ever the same circumstances arose again, I would not repeat what I had done. Over the next few days her condition improved; despite her having collapsed lungs, difficulty in breathing and a suspected heart attack.

The hospital staff had started decorating the ward in preparation for Christmas, which was ten days away. On 15 December all the drips and drain tubes were removed and Chris was making good progress. A histology report showed that tissue removed for biopsy revealed no evidence of a tumour being present. However three days later a supplementary report showed that further slides treated with immunological stains demonstrated the presence of residual, poorly differentiated carcinoma both in the posterior wall of the bladder and in the kidneys. The cancer was still evident, regardless of the total pelvic clearance, which had aimed to remove it surgically.

Chris continued to receive a mixture of drugs daily and she became very dependent on morphine to ease her pain.

On December 25th we spent our Christmas together in Ward One. Chris had managed to get one of her friends to do her Christmas shopping and she surprised Rebecca and me with presents. Mine was a set of skiing equipment; Rebecca had a rocking horse and some small gifts. We had bought Chris a new dressing gown, slippers, undergarments, and a small three inch screen LCD television, so that she would not miss any of her favourite programmes when she was to unable to leave her bed.

Four weeks passed before Chris was discharged on 23 January. During this time she was referred to a hospital psychiatrist because of an addiction to 'slow release' morphine. She had become dependent on four milligrams each day. Thankfully he was able to help and a few days later she was able to cope with smaller doses.

On 31 January, 1990, she was re-admitted to Princess Alexandra's Hospital. She had spent only a week at home, during which time she encountered several bouts of vomiting and suffered severe abdominal pains; her colostomy had not been functioning properly for ten days, the equivalent to being constipated.

An external examination of her abdomen found it to be soft with no obvious abnormalities. An intravenous infusion was started and a feeding tube was passed into Chris's stomach via her nose.

On 1 February, twelve months to the day since her first admission for the D and C, Chris was still having some gripping pains in her abdomen and she was taken into theatre for examination under anaesthesia. Soft faecal matter was felt in the colostomy. Drip-feeding was again commenced and she remained on nutritional fluids until 5 February, when she was able to start a light diet.

On 12 February, her thirty-fifth birthday, Chris's nasal feeding tube was removed. She still had bouts of nausea from an upset stomach. It was decided that a further investigative laparotomy would be necessary and this was performed two days later. It revealed marked adhesions and a grossly dilated bowel though there was no obvious spread of secondary cancer. When the small bowel was freed, a stricture in the terminal ileum was noted. There were several small perforations, which were repaired. This was quite substantial surgery, in an area of the body that is very susceptible to pain: an epidural anaesthetic was placed in Chris's chest to control it.

Once again she encountered a prolonged and difficult recovery period over the following several weeks. She experienced periods of fever. At one point the central venous line had to be removed and when it was tested it showed the presence of a fever- causing bacterium. Because of the partial hysterectomy, Dr Baxendall prescribed hormone replacement therapy (HRT). Chris now began sticking Estraderm patches on her left thigh.

The histology report on the bowel removed during the total pelvic clearance operation showed no evidence of tumour or of radiation damage. On 8 March a CT scan showed an abscess, measuring approximately 10 x 6 x 5 cm, which extended from the lower margin of the liver to the pelvis. Two attempts were made to drain this, the second of which was successful, on 8 March. Five days later, a large catheter was inserted and a further fifty millilitres of thick dark blood was aspirated. This aspiration was instituted twice daily until 16 March. An ultrasound examination then revealed that the abscess was resolving but another problem followed: several gallstones were found in the gall bladder and bile duct.

Chris was discharged from hospital shortly afterwards and an appointment for visual exploration of the bile duct, pancreas and liver was arranged, which was to take place in the nearby NHS Princess Margaret's Hospital in Swindon. On 3 April a large stone was removed from the common bile duct; the smaller stones passed spontaneously and there were no complications.

FIFTEEN

A wonderful respite

Chris was now 'officially' discharged from Princess Alexandra's Hospital in Wroughton. However she was to return on more than one occasion with further complications. Except for occasional days at home, she had spent a total of fourteen months receiving hospital care.

Her condition at this point was recorded during an outpatient appointment on 10 May. The report read:

She still complains of some vaginal discharge, which is intermittently bloodstained. An examination of the vulva and introitus are well oestrogenised, the vagina is about two inches long and surrounded by solid tissue, which is recurrence of tumour, or inflammatory, or post-radiation fibrosis. She will not be able to have sexual intercourse without surgical extension of the vagina. At present her body image prevents any sexual contact. She should continue using Estraderm patches and will be seen again in two months.

On the evening of 18 May I had a frank discussion with Chris. Neither of us knew how long she would live but her quality of life now seemed at its lowest yet. She was unable to eat properly and her sleep pattern was totally irregular. She would often catch up on lost sleep during the day. The plethora of medications she took included anti-nausea drugs, morphine in solid and fluid form for pain relief and vitamin supplements. The district nurse attended on a daily basis and there were regular visits from her GP. Chris needed help each time she moved around the house. It seemed apparent that her life expectancy would be short.

It was decided that I would become her main carer and would resign from my position as assistant manager at the Anchor Foods Dairy Company. I would finish work on 30 July. Fortunately, before this date I was made redundant and the money I received, together with our mortgage protection insurance, gave us enough financial security for the year. At least now Chris was able to enjoy more time with Rebecca, despite her illness. She had already missed so much of her baby's development.

A letter from the Director of Social Services confirmed that her employment as Officer-in-Charge of The Cedars Residential Home for the Elderly was being terminated, on the grounds of permanent ill health, effective from January, 1990. It also stated that residents and colleagues would sadly miss her and thanked her for the invaluable service she had given since she joined. Ironically, they wished her good health.

Chris was medically pensioned off from her employment with Wiltshire Social Services. Her short career had come to an end. She was disappointed to have received this news but it finally clarified her position.

During July Chris was still complaining of a bloodstained vaginal discharge, which often smelled offensive. Her symptoms seemed to suggest a recurrence of the cancer in the vaginal vault. As she could only be treated symptomatically, antiseptic dressings were prescribed. Her next outpatient appointment was not until October, but on 20 August she was admitted to hospital again because of several heavy vaginal bleeding episodes. These had been periodic since her last appointment. She was admitted to theatre later that day and three biopsies were taken from the pelvic mass. A vaginal pack was inserted. Three days later, the results from the biopsies showed only fibrosis and some inflammatory change. The vaginal pack was removed and she was discharged on 24 August.

During an outpatient appointment on September 6, an examination by Dr Baxendall revealed that there was still some discharge but the bleeding had now stopped. Another appointment was arranged for the following month. Twelve days later, on 18

September, she was once again admitted, this time as an emergency case.

Severe abdominal pains had always caused great concern and had necessitated Chris's frequent admissions to hospital. The cause this time was an attack of inflammation in the gall bladder. Following treatment, she was discharged on 25 September only to be readmitted on 5 October. On 8 October she underwent a routine surgical removal of the gall bladder. She was discharged again five days later.

After that period in hospital Chris began to feel better. Her strength was recovering slowly as the days went on. A few months earlier in July, we had made plans to go abroad on holiday for a while. It was provisionally booked through the tour operator for November but those plans had looked so very doubtful so many times that I really did not believe they would materialise. Now the holiday date was drawing near and we extended our original two-week break on the Greek side of Cyprus to six months. It was Chris who thought of the idea, because if we self-catered for that period it would only be slightly more expensive than the original two-week holiday.

I arranged to rent out our house through a letting agent. An Australian family was to take up residence. The house would remain fully furnished except for some of our personal belongings, which we stored in the attic. We would have until April 1991 to reassess our lives, everything depending, of course, on the state of Christine's health. The current prognosis looked somewhat bleak but there were now some encouraging signs that the disease was not recurring and at least she was now well enough to travel. We hoped the change of scenery and the warm climate would help to improve her recovery. At worst, if her condition deteriorated it would hardly matter at this stage. We did what we thought was best.

Dr Baxendall sanctioned the travel arrangements. On 19

November, two days before we left for Cyprus, he examined Chris at the gynaecology clinic. Her vaginal discharge seemed to be improving. He handed her a typed letter to take with her, addressed to a consultant gynaecologist in Cyprus. It would facilitate her access to hospital if necessary and was a comforting reassurance. If she developed any complications requiring medical assistance, she could be treated at the Royal Air Force Base Hospital in Akrotiri.

Chris left the clinic feeling more optimistic, particularly after reading the contents of Dr Baxendall's letter:

MRS CHRISTINE LUCEY

This lady had carcinoma of the cervix diagnosed in May 1989. Since then she has had the uterus, bladder, and lower bowel removed – December 1989, X-ray therapy and chemotherapy. There is considerable induration and necrosis in the pelvis causing a vaginal discharge, but biopsy of the vaginal region on 22 08 90, showed no recurrence of disease. She had her gall bladder removed 08 10 90.

If she needs medical attention please see.

We arrived in Limassol on 21 November, 1990. The hotel and its complex, including our adjoining apartment, were perfect. An added bonus for this chosen haven was the seclusion of the resort. There were fewer guests than we had expected, which allowed us to enjoy more privacy. Gone now were the hordes of foreign tourists, the crowds of energetic and excited young people who were often found running amok and causing mayhem. It was the ideal opportunity for our long retreat. The island was ours to savour and enjoy at our leisure. It seemed that we had the whole of Cyprus to ourselves.

The ground floor apartment, that was to be our new home for the next six months had only three small steps, with a bannister, that separated the two levels. The lounge, dining area and kitchen were on the lower level; the bathroom, bedroom with two single beds and balcony were on the upper. Chris and Rebecca quickly commandeered the two beds; I settled for the sofa.

Our first morning began with an unusual adventure. A small earthquake shook the apartment. The tremor caused the settee on which I was sleeping to move slightly. It was enough to wake us all up. Later we learnt that this was a regular occurrence. We were happy as long as the tremors remained small. The incident did not deter us from enjoying ourselves and we wasted no time in hiring a car to explore the island.

We spent many a long day on the various magnificent beaches. Chris would sunbathe cautiously, exposing only the lower parts of her legs. The temperature was comfortable, averaging twenty-three degrees. We had picnics on the isolated golden sands and watched the cruise liners and ships of all descriptions sailing serenely past. We paddled in the beautiful warm blue waters of the Mediterranean and Rebecca built endless sandcastles, pausing only to run to the water's edge in order to collect small plastic buckets of water. This she would use to fill the moat that she had meticulously scraped out with her tiny spade. Her constructions stood alone. Unchallenged.

It was a different world. The English winter seemed so far away. We soon became accustomed to the Greek Cypriot way of life and it was therapeutic for all of us. Chris seemed like a different woman. It was hard to believe that she had been to hell and back for almost two years. Now she was almost her old self, beginning to laugh again, singing nursery songs, playing games with Rebecca and holding her hand tightly everywhere we went. The stress and anxiety was melting away under the warmth of the Cypriot sun.

Chris was getting stronger every day. She looked better than I had seen her look for years. She was eating well at last, enjoying the abundance of fresh fruit that was available and meals at tavernas in the lovely mountain villages. We drove around the island, enjoying its beautiful landscape, both of us enjoying

Rebecca. I felt glad that we were operating like a real family again, even though we were divided by Chris's disability and the emotional scars her experience had left on both of us.

We met new friends every day, other holidaymakers and local residents. We went out sometimes with a group of army nurses that we met. They had been posted to Cyprus and knew Chris from RAF Wroughton. We also visited some new friends who owned a small villa in the village of Anoyira and they shared their hospitality with us and their knowledge of the local culture. In turn they introduced us to their friends, mainly Greek families. We were privileged to become a special part of their way of life.

We put the last fourteen months behind us, with its nightmare of endless hospital treatments. We lived for the day and secretly hoped for a permanent recovery. But it was not to last.

Regrettably, the threat of war in the Gulf brought an unexpected end to our long-term holiday. Our plans to stay until April had to be abandoned and we arrived home in England on 16 January, 1991. The Foreign Office had issued a warning, recommending that all British tourists should leave Cyprus. Iraq had begun its invasion of Kuwait and the British Armed Forces were about to assist its allies in liberating the country from the grip of the ruthless dictatorship of Iraq's president, Saddam Hussein.

Fortunately for us, the family that had taken temporary residence in our home had decided to return early to Australia and we were able to move back into our house on 17 January, the day the Gulf War started.

Sixteen

I think you should get your smear tests checked

On 28 February, the consultant radiotherapist at Princess Margaret Hospital, Swindon, who was collecting data on patients treated at Oxford, wrote to Dr Baxendall asking for details on Chris's progress.

Chris attended the outpatient department at Princess Alexandra's Hospital on 14 March. She still had a vaginal discharge with some bleeding, but had gained weight and now weighed eight and a half stone. On examination, the pelvis was solid with a narrow vagina. The rectum was tender with bright red bleeding. Dr Baxendall told her that he would contact the radiotherapist at Princess Margaret's Hospital, inform him of the current vaginal discharge and find out if there was a possibility of further radiotherapy. He received a reply that simply stated the radiotherapist had no suggestions to make.

It was early April and I had now been off work for almost nine months. Chris was becoming more independent around the house and enjoyed spending time in the kitchen preparing meals. Usually, Rebecca was nearby; she especially liked mixing ingredients for cakes or anything to do with baking. She would stand on a chair near the kitchen table or work surface, wearing an apron that Chris had folded several times around her small waist. She was always holding a wooden spoon in her hand and if she wasn't whisking the cake mix, she was licking it from the spoon.

There was a lull in Chris's treatment. It appeared that the doctors were simply waiting to see what happened next. Chris continued to have CT scans, usually every three months but they showed no evidence of tumour recurrence. Her only real discomfort was the vaginal and rectal discharge. She was coping well with her stomas and the daily regimen of medication and vitamin supplements.

Psychologically, she was approaching life with newfound strength and determination, fighting the incredible severity of her illness every step of the way. The holiday in Cyprus had helped tremendously. Chris told me that she wanted to live long enough to watch Rebecca start school. This alone would keep her going.

One evening we discussed the idea of my returning to work. Chris felt that it would be a positive move, as she could now manage better on her own. I was not sure what employment to pursue. I was reluctant to go back to a managerial position or any mundane nine-to-five job. I telephoned my friend, Alan, who was a police officer, as the idea of joining the service had crossed my mind a few years earlier; but at thirty-nine, had I left it too late? He gave me details of the recruiting process, and the following day I made enquires.

I passed the initial entrance exam and the three-day Selection Board in May. On 23 September, 1991, I was officially recruited and on my way to the Police Training College at Chantmarle in Dorset to start my new career as a constable in the Wiltshire Constabulary. I usually travelled to the college on Monday mornings with three other raw recruits, returning home on Friday afternoon. I hated being away and longed for the day when I would see some real police action. The teaching techniques at Chantmarle seemed better suited to kindergarten children. I could not get used to pulling up my beanbag, the group-orientated method of learning, or to the silly role-playing. But like everything in life you either accept it or you leave. I accepted it.

Chris attended the clinic for assessment on 18 November. Her weight was recorded at nine stone. She still had a vaginal discharge, for which nothing could be done. An internal examination showed that the vagina was definitive. Her sex life was still nonexistent.

She was seen again by the surgeons at the Princess Alexandra Hospital in their clinic on 27 November. The hospital records showed that there were some worrying features: she complained of low back pain extending down both thighs, with occasional loin pain. A further

CT scan was arranged. The result from the scan, taken on 5 December, showed no recurrence of tumour, although there was a 2.5 cm cyst at the apex of the rectal stump. She was reviewed again on December 11 and was reassured by the gynaecologist.

Three months later, on 11 March, 1992, she was examined by another specialist at the hospital, who was the Cade Professor of Surgery and Adviser in Urology. His findings were:

> *The pain in her perineum was radiating to the right buttock and had become more pronounced. She had noticed a loss of mucus rectally. I suspect that her tumour has recurred, but feel that there is little in the way of treatment that can be offered.*

He arranged a further appointment for April and told her that he would discuss her future management with Air Commodore Baxendall. It was possible that she would be admitted for examination under anaesthesia.

Two days later, I completed my police training. Chris and Rebecca travelled to Chantmarle with our close friends, Alan and Teresa, to watch the final ceremonial parade that was the culmination of the twenty-week course, plus several weeks training at Wiltshire Police Headquarters. This was an achievement for all of the recruits. I continued training with my probationary period in Swindon. Eighteen months of general police duties remained.

Shortly before Chris returned for her appointment in April, she received a telephone call from a friend who was also a nurse and worked at the local hospital. She knew the circumstances surrounding Chris's illness and had somehow discovered that one of her smears, taken in 1988 was suspicious. "Chris," she said, "I've just found out something. I think you should get your smear tests checked. One might be positive!" The initial jolt of hearing those words came as a tremendous shock. Chris couldn't believe that there could be anything wrong with the smears, she trusted the doctors implicitly and found it hard to imagine that they could make such a blunder.

She told me about the phone call and asked me whether I thought she should have the tests re-checked? I was slightly apprehensive too, thinking her friend must be mistaken. Chris had explained the procedure involving smear tests and it was difficult to imagine any flaws in hospital procedures. I suggested a telephone call to a solicitor to seek advice.

Chris waited for three days before finally convincing herself that she did have some doubts about the professionalism of the medical fraternity, including one doctor whom she trusted and respected, Air Commodore Baxendall. She contacted a firm of solicitors in Devizes and discussed the vague contents of her friend's telephone conversation with John Anton Czul, a specialist in medical negligence. His fees at the onset almost deterred us from pursuing the matter. His rate was a hundred pounds per hour. We were advised that if there was genuine litigation in respect of neglectful smear sampling, Chris might be entitled to Legal Aid, but we would have to pay the fees first. Nonetheless, we asked him to start the proceedings.

Luckily, Chris had kept her own record of monthly periods since her miscarriage in 1984 and this also recorded her hospital treatment, from pregnancy in 1987, right up until 1992. She began by submitting a short handwritten statement to the solicitor. Two weeks later, she completed a detailed seventeen-page testimony disclosing every medical event that had occurred during those five years.

The long process of legal investigation, instigated on the basis of that one telephone call, had started.

SEVENTEEN

Nothing more can be done for you

On April 3, 1992, Chris was seen again at the gynaecology clinic. Her symptoms remained the same, with a twenty-four-hour history of copious vaginal discharge, coupled with back and vaginal pain. She was too sore to be examined and was told to return in three days.

Rebecca had started playgroup in the local evangelical church, which was only a short distance from our home. The day before Chris's next hospital visit was due, she decided to stay and help the nursery teacher but began to feel unwell, experiencing the feeling of something 'dropping' inside her abdomen. She left the playgroup with Rebecca and telephoned Dr Baxendall on arriving home. When she explained her symptoms she was told to come straight to the hospital. Luckily I had finished work early that day and I was able to take her. She was taken to theatre for examination under anaesthesia: Dr Baxendall and the urologist performed the operation, during which biopsies were taken.

These were subsequently reported to show 'poorly differentiated carcinoma indistinguishable from the original cervical biopsies'. On 11 April a further laparotomy was performed, when it was discovered that the terminal ileum and caecum were involved with a *malignant* abscess, which was removed. The apex of the rectal stump and the vagina were amputated along with the malignant tissue. An apron of abdominal fatty tissue segment was freed and laid over the raw area.

Considering the extent of this surgery, Chris's postoperative condition was excellent. The dropping feeling that she had experienced had been due to a rupturing of her bowel, allowing faecal matter to drain through her vaginal cavity. This had resulted in extreme pain. Chris was told that a growth the size of a grapefruit had been removed. Her worst fears were now realised: the cancer had spread. The surgeon also disclosed that there were now so many abdominal areas with cancerous growths that nothing more could be done for her.

On 14 April Chris received two units of blood and her vaginal pack was removed the following day under general anaesthesia. She was feeling better and more comfortable but she had a low-grade fever. Her colostomy was now working properly and she was discharged from hospital on 21 April.

It was to be her last operation at Princess Alexandra Hospital. No other surgery was possible. The surgeon wrote to inform the consultant oncologist, Dr A C Jones, of the operation that he had performed, describing the malignant pelvic abscess involving the terminal ileum and caecum. He enclosed a copy of the histology of the tissue removed during the operation and requested the oncologist's advice regarding the possibility of any further therapy. The tissue from the vaginal wall, the small bowel and the tumour associated with the rectum all contained poorly differentiated invasive carcinoma.

Chris attended Dr Jones's clinic at Princess Margaret Hospital on 18 May. I sat with her as she waited to see the consultant oncologist, to learn whether she could continue with further chemotherapy. She was very anxious. Ironically she was reasonably fit at this time, her vaginal discharge had largely resolved following the operation of 11 April. Jones examined her in the clinic and recommended two scans which would check her renal function and blood count. He would then decide whether to arrange another course of chemotherapy.

On leaving the hospital we discussed this possible option. I was not convinced that the horrific bouts of nausea, vomiting and loss of appetite were worth it, especially when there was no guarantee that it would cure her disease. Chris said that she would find it almost impossible to tolerate the degree of suffering she had experienced before. Yet, if the therapy became available, she felt she had no choice. The surgeon who had performed her last operation had told her that if any treatment were offered, then she should take it.

Memories of what had happened after Chris's earlier treatment, all of the surgery and the fact that she had nearly died on two occasions, were still fresh in my mind. I urged her to consider her remaining quality of life, saying that I felt she should *enjoy* whatever time she had left to live. She reminded me that they were now using a new anti-sickness drug to alleviate the dreadful side effects of chemotherapy, apparently with good results. The symptoms would be nowhere near as bad as they were before. In the end I said it was her decision. She knew that I would give my total support to whatever she decided.

Chris decided to have more chemotherapy and returned to see Dr Jones in Oxford on 8 June. He recommended six courses of treatment to be administered over a period of six months. Her admission was deferred until 18 June.

Chris was radiant, her general health was good and she had recovered from the depression that followed being told that her cancer had spread and nothing else could be done for her. She still had hopes that the treatment would help her to live and she continued to maintain a positive outlook. Later she would make enquires regarding homeopathic medicines and spiritual healing.

A conservatory was built onto the back of our house so that Chris could spend hours relaxing there, looking out onto the garden, enjoying quiet moments of meditation. It allowed her some privacy and became her sanctuary of peace and tranquillity. Her many friends and former colleagues continued to visit and they sat together in the comfort of this separate annex, drinking tea as they reminisced. Rebecca knew that it was Mummy's special room and she respected the times Chris wanted to be alone.

Chris would drive Rebecca to nursery each morning and collect her at noon. I continued to work my varied pattern of shifts: days, evenings and night duties. Our lifestyle had once more begun to return to normality.

Chris's first course of chemotherapy commenced on 18 June. The routine of travelling to the Churchill Hospital in Oxford had started again. She was discharged on 22 June in spite of being nauseated. On the 23rd she was readmitted with uncontrollable nausea, vomiting, abdominal pain and headache but her symptoms settled and she was discharged again on the 25th. We did not know whether the new anti-sickness drug was working at all.

Results from a blood test taken on 6 July at Princess Margaret's Hospital in Swindon indicated that Chris's white cell count, haemoglobin and platelets were all satisfactory. An adjustment to the second pulse of treatment, due at this time, was now suggested because her vaginal discharge had started again. She had also developed tinnitus, noises in the ear, as a result of the first course of chemotherapy.

Chris had another blood count check on Monday, 13 July, then she was admitted on the 16th for the second course of treatment. Her tinnitus had improved slightly and she was keen to continue despite her severe sickness. Each course was supposed to last for three days and I arrived at the hospital to bring her home on the morning of 19 July. I walked into Ward Seven, the same one in which she began her therapy three years ago in 1989. She occupied the first bed on the left and was sitting on its edge. As I approached she looked up at me, appearing tired and lethargic.

"Good morning, darling. How are you today?" I said.

"Who are you?" she replied.

I sat next to her, thinking she was being humorous. "I'm Don, remember? Your husband."

She stared at me as if I was a total stranger. Her eyes seemed distant and I realised that there was something awfully wrong, "You're not my husband. You're the doctor, aren't you?"

I called a nurse. She sat next to Chris and began talking gently to her but she could make little sense of what Chris said. The nurse called the Senior House Officer, explaining that Chris had told her she was feeling dopey and dizzy. He observed that she was totally disorientated and thought she had reacted badly to one of the anti-cancer drugs. She was kept in the ward that day and reviewed later in the evening.

The following day she had not completely recovered but was much improved. Dr Jones saw her on his daily ward round and discussed the next session of chemotherapy. No mention was made of her reaction, except that they would reduce the dose of Ifosfamide on her third course of treatment. She was discharged on 22 July, the day of our fourteenth wedding anniversary.

The treatment continued the following month, when a CT body scan proved disappointing. It was difficult to interpret but suggested the possibility of progressive disease. We decided to consult with Jones regarding the outcome of the chemotherapy treatment and whether it was worthwhile continuing. Three sessions remained and it was decided to review the scan results.

On 10 September, Chris informed Dr Jones that she did not want to continue with the chemotherapy. Together we had come to the conclusion that it was having no effect in stopping the disease and she had now realised that her quality of life was far more important than having to endure further anguish which would, more than likely, prove to be all for nothing. It was agreed that she would continue having CT scans every three months to monitor the progression of the disease.

EIGHTEEN

Recorded Statement of the Facts

Rebecca was now four and a half years old and had started infant school in September. Chris had got her wish that she would live long enough to see the day. She was able to take her to school and often helped in the classroom, just as she had at the nursery, astounding everyone with her determination to lead a normal life, like any ordinary healthy young woman. The one exception to this 'normality' was the tremendous toll that Chris's illness had taken on the intimate side of our relationship.

On 10 December the outcome of a CT scan showed no further progression of the disease. The end of another year was near and only one appointment had taken place with the solicitor who would ultimately become the driving force behind the future legal battle. Although the wheels were in motion, it was to be some time before there were any developments resulting from the suspected 'positive' smear sample.

At the start of 1993 Chris began having spiritual healing sessions at home. I never quite understood the technique or the logic used by the healer. It was something that Chris kept confidential and I endorsed her preference for privacy. She once tried to explain the methodology and theory of her newfound therapy to me. It involved meditation and relaxation, practised while listening to tapes of calming music, birdsong, waterfalls and surf breaking gently on the seashore. The healer would then place her hands on top of Chris's head for a short period, which was intended to help in ridding the cancer from her body. I have to say that I was sceptical about its effectiveness but all that mattered was that Chris believed in it.

Another further CT scan in March still showed no change in the progression of the cancer. This good news encouraged Chris to become even more positive. Her hair, totally lost during the last session of chemotherapy, was now starting to grow back again. The NHS wig, which Chris had worn for months, was cast aside, never to be worn again.

I had now completed eighteen months of my probationary training period in the police force and I volunteered for response car duties in the town of Cricklade in the rural area of Wiltshire. It was close to our home and gave me the opportunity to call in to see Chris and Rebecca occasionally during shifts. The constabulary had shown compassion and understanding towards our welfare throughout my early service and my friends and colleagues gave enormous and unrelenting support to all of us.

On March 12, 1993, the first letter arrived from our solicitor. The slow and lengthy legal wrangle had begun. For anyone who has never been involved in a lawsuit, beware of the potential complexities. It can cause apprehension, disappointment and frustration. It is generally very stressful and takes an inordinate length of time. However, if the evidence is strong enough against the opposition, this is all you need.

The legal process can cost large sums of money. Since we had to rely solely on my income, this was a worrying time for us. As our personal insurance policy did not include any legal protection cover, we hoped the Legal Aid Board would approve funding for the potential litigation.

This first letter from the solicitors had contained forms explaining their terms and conditions of business and a standing order to be completed for my bank. These were signed and returned. We had now committed ourselves to the substantial £100 hourly legal fees. It was the beginning of reams of correspondence and numerous solicitors' appointments that would gather momentum as time moved on. We waited patiently to hear if our application for legal aid had been accepted.

In April, 1993, the solicitor suggested that we should provide a videotape depicting our lifestyle, relating in particular how the effects of the disease had caused Chris so much physical and psychological pain. Its contents would include a statement explaining how she had become affected emotionally and mentally by the abrupt end of our physical relationship.

This videotaped affidavit was to be held by the solicitor should it be required to be used in evidence. Chris knew that the reasoning behind the request was that she would probably not still be alive if the case eventually went to court.

Chris began the interview with her personal details, family background and her education and employment history. She explained how we met, our marriage, careers and social activities and the birth of Rebecca. We had enjoyed a good life, with two or three holidays a year. Once we had a new baby to enjoy as well, it seemed that life could hardly get better. Now her quality of life was very poor. She had little time to herself since she was too unwell to be left alone. By the evening of every day she was exhausted and in pain.

Then she talked in detail about her health care and the disappointment of learning the history of her misdiagnosed smears. She explained how Air Commodore Baxendall had been worried about the abnormal feel of her cervix when she was carrying Rebecca, felt that it would not dilate and had recommended a Caesarean delivery. She made reference to her non-referral to a colposcopy clinic after the birth and how this had subsequently reduced her chances of living a normal life.

She described her present state of health and prognosis and how impossible it was for her to have an intimate relationship. Not only was it now physically impossible, but also the mental and emotional scars she bore made it inconceivable. At this point she became too distressed to continue discussing the subject and spoke of other matters, including her lack of counselling throughout her ordeal. She had never felt like talking to anyone about her illness since the time that the nurse had reduced her confidence when she had been worried the doctors might think her cancer was the result of promiscuity.

She ended her statement by commenting that she had confounded all of her doctors' expectations by surviving so long. She was generally regarded by the medics as a walking miracle. But now there was nothing more they could do to help her.

"We shall have to wait and see how things go," she concluded.

NINETEEN

Failure to diagnose cancer

Without any adverse treatment effects Chris's general well-being had improved noticeably. She was beginning to have a better sleep pattern, with fewer visits to the bathroom to empty the colostomy and urostomy bags. Both stomas were functioning satisfactorily and there were no prolonged complications.

Chris's newfound supply of energy inspired her with the confidence to socialise more and her appearance improved to the point where she began wearing smartly fitting clothes again, spending less time in nightwear or tracksuits. She wanted to achieve as much as possible in whatever time she had left.

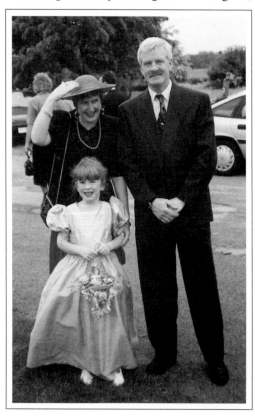

In early spring, we were able to have a few days away on the Isle of Wight and were guests at a friend's wedding in May. Our social life was improving and we began to go out more often as a family. Chris enjoyed taking Rebecca swimming. She wore a special bathing costume that discreetly covered her abdominal stomas. They went for frequent walks in the park. Here at last was the sort of relationship between a mother and daughter. They were inseparable.

Chris and Rebecca went to Durham to stay with her family for two weeks in the summer of that year, while I continued to work. On their return home, Chris started attending the Royal London Homeopathic Hospital NHS Trust and began a course of alternative medication that was available to help control the vicious cycle of pain, disability and depression. GPs, who are very much aware of what terminal patients go through, are usually sympathetic towards complementary therapies of many kinds. Approval for Chris to attend was authorised by the local District Health Authority and the homeopathic remedies she was prescribed were Thuja, Iscador and Mistletoe.

In September I completed my two-year police probationary period and applied to become an Authorised Firearms Officer. Their shift pattern was different to my regular hours, consisting of four day's duty alternating with four days off. This would allow me more time with my family. A firearms course was due to start in early 1994. I awaited the outcome of my application to join.

Meanwhile other domestic matters were unfolding at home. Our ex-childminder, 'Nanny' Jean, was concerned that she had not seen Rebecca for some time, though she would occasionally visit Chris, she always seemed to miss Rebecca and wanted to keep in touch. Jean's employment had come to an end when Chris became well enough to care for Rebecca herself, but she had offered to help again if ever we needed her. I thought the time was right and soon afterwards Jean was re-employed, helping with the housework and babysitting. Thus I was reprieved and Jean would continue to stay in contact with Rebecca indefinitely.

Good news had also arrived from our legal representatives, the application for legal aid had been granted. We were even to be refunded the expenditure from earlier appointments with our lawyer, except that a percentage of the funds made available by the Legal Aid Board had to be repaid, which equated to two hundred pounds. But this was negligible compared to the possible settlement amounts being mentioned.

The personal injury section on page four of the form described the details of Injury:

MEDICAL NEGLIGENCE CASE:

Failure to diagnose cancer, in early course resulted in, hysterectomy, colostomy, urostomy, and ultimately total abdominal clearance, acute physical pain, and psychological distress, date when first sustained: 01 05 89.

To help support the claim, our solicitor had obtained medical records covering a period of approximately twenty years or so from the hospitals and general practitioners who had been responsible for the management of Christine's medical care. Soon, definite proof of the misreported smear tests was to be confirmed by one of the medical experts. This would provide the essential evidence necessary to prepare for the long legal battle.

An expert witness had also been contacted to provide assistance with the inquiry. He was Pat Soutter, MD, Reader in Gynaecological Oncology at Hammersmith Hospital, London. We now had two experts researching the various aspects of Chris's medical care. They would establish the veracity of the written statement Chris had provided as evidence to Mr Czul. Both would play a crucial role in preparing medico-legal reports regarding the allegations that we made against the defendants.

The true extent of the blunders relating to the misreporting of Chris's smear tests was revealed following a meeting with our solicitor on 6 November, 1993. Our second expert, Professor Roger Cotton, produced a report relating his findings when he attended the Pathology Department at Princess Margaret's Hospital, Swindon, on October 15, 1993. There he examined several cervical smears that disclosed, not only shocking evidence of numerous misreported samples but also mismanagement of patient care in the eleven years from 1977 to 1988. Even more disturbing was the smear result of June, 1988. This was one of many smears that were taken during Chris's extensive period of postnatal bleeding and which she had been told was negative. The smear test had not only been under-reported to the GP by the Cytology Department at Princess Margaret's Hospital but also was missed by Dr Baxendall, the consultant gynaecologist for seven and a half months, allowing time for aggressive and swift progression of the tumour in her cervix. This smear test had been grossly under-reported due to serious misinterpretation of abnormal cells present, suggesting that a repeat smear in one year was all that was necessary. This smear was actually frankly 'positive' containing numerous obvious cancer cells. Professor Cotton's report contained proof that substantiated the allegation originally made by Chris's nursing friend at Princess Margaret's Hospital. There had indeed been a 'positive' smear but it had been missed.

The defendants that were soon to be issued with a writ were:

(1) Swindon Health Authority, Cytology Department, now known as Swindon and Marlborough Hospitals National Health Service Trust, for their part in failing to notice or act in providing a proper standard of care, on several counts.

(2) The Secretary of State for Defence, acting on behalf of Dr Baxendall and others, for their part in several counts of negligence.

TWENTY

Our marriage was in ruins

Towards the end of November, something happened to temporarily shift the concern from Chris to me. No two days are the same in the life of an active police officer. This particular day indicated just how unpredictable things could get.

It began with the usual hour of desk duty at the station in Cricklade, catching up with the masses of paperwork that all police officers loathe. After this, it was time for vehicle patrol duties; out in the car attending numerous incidents including 'domestics', sudden deaths, suicides, road traffic offences and accidents, to name but a few.

My first enquiry concerned a 'misper', the term for a missing person. I was asked to go the village of Purton, to Bentham House, an institute for mentally disturbed patients. A phone call from a member of staff there had reported that the man in question had left the home on several occasions and had returned after a while. However this time there was no sign of him and they were genuinely concerned for his safety. He had been away for several hours. I was unable to obtain a precise description of his clothing or any distinguishing features. I knew only that he was twenty-five years old and taking medication. The staff thought that he might have tried to walk the six miles to Swindon to visit his mother.

Before attending the home to obtain further details, I had to refuel the near-empty police vehicle. I drove to the local services on the A419, near the town of Cricklade. There I spotted a man acting suspiciously. He was sitting on the protective barrier near the roadside and tapping the metal surface with what appeared to be a thin white stick. It occurred to me that he fitted the less-than-perfect description of the 'misper' from Bentham House. I was in uniform and when I approached him he made a run for it across the busy dual carriageway. He clambered over a gate into a field. I chased after him and quickly caught up, at which point he lunged at me with a five-foot pole with a sharpened metal point, stabbing my left eye and hand.

I had lost the vision in one eye and the other had partially glazed over by the time I managed to climb over a gate and flee back to the garage where I called for backup from Swindon. The 'troops' arrived and a police dog handler and her dog caught 'the bad guy'. I was whisked off to hospital in an ambulance where I received treatment and was subjected to a barrage of eye tests. I was discharged after a few hours but the eye tests continued for several weeks afterwards.

I remember telephoning Chris from the hospital that night, to tell her that I had been involved in a slight altercation on the A419 and that the media were all over the hospital trying to get news coverage. I told her to watch the nine o'clock news but not to worry because I was fine and would be home as soon as possible. As it happened, I returned in time to watch the news myself with Chris and Rebecca. The injury was less severe than everyone had first imagined, although my eye was swollen, closed over and bruised and I was unable to continue with my duties for six weeks.

The twenty-five-year-old man was convicted of causing 'Actual Bodily Harm' and was detained in a secure unit where he was able to receive better care and attention for his illness than at Bentham House.

There were more visits than usual to our house during those six weeks and I received a number of phone calls and considerable correspondence from friends, colleagues and the general public.

I returned to work shortly after Christmas with no eye or hand complications. The incident unsettled me and made me realise that I, too, was vulnerable to incapacitation. In short, it made me all too aware of my own mortality. Nonetheless I did gain some comfort, knowing that there were people who were prepared to show *me* some concern for a change. It may seem selfish but I had been on the sidelines for four years, while Chris had received all of the attention. I had done the caring, nursing, helping, feeding, bathing, running around, shopping, working, talking, listening and had given support, support, support, day in, day out, there was never a let-up even on our so-called holidays. It had to take an injury before people understood that I needed support too.

It had never occurred to me to feel sorry for myself while Chris was suffering so much. All I thought of was her ordeal. I prepared myself for the worst on those occasions when she nearly died and looked on in despair as her quality of life deteriorated so drastically. Throughout those awful times I watched as she sank lower and lower, until she had become a completely different person from the attractive, healthy and vibrant young woman I had once known.

Now though, Chris was well. She seemed almost on the point of recovery but she was still unable to have any intimate contact with me, no form of sexual activity at all. We never even kissed any more. Gone were the warm embraces, the loving hugs. Instead we would exchange the occasional peck on the cheek. In effect, our marriage was in ruins, non-existent. We were little more than just good friends, though we were still happy as a family. We both doted on our precious daughter, Rebecca and we knew that she was the reason that kept us together. We continued to sleep in separate bedrooms, Chris still sharing our bed with Rebecca.

Chris had started taking steroids, which had the effect of making her look bloated, and her weight was approaching eleven stone. I was beginning to believe that the cancer was well and truly in remission and that she would survive for quite some time and live a relatively normal life. But I knew that the woman that I had married and loved was anything but the same woman. I still loved her but it was a different kind of love. It was as if she had been taken from me and turned into a monster. How were we meant to stay the same after all that had happened?

Deep down inside me, I knew in my heart that I could never leave her for someone else. I empathised with Chris's suffering. It was not her fault that she was how she was now. Though at times I secretly longed to hold another woman in my arms, to have someone healthy to kiss and to embrace and with whom to have sexual pleasure. I was, after all, still a young man.

Chris, sweet lady that she was, would sometimes encourage me to leave her, for my own sake. Yet I knew that at other times she was also very jealous of me, jealous because I still had my health and could do anything I wanted to do. She had become more and more independent since suspending her conventional therapy and the latest CT scans indicated that there was no progression in the tumour. I was pleased that she had reached this stage, even though she was still consuming vast amounts of medication each day.

Twenty-One

The holiday of a lifetime

The first six months of 1994 brought about many changes. I completed my course and became an Authorised Firearms Officer employed on security operations within the Wiltshire Constabulary. My duties involved armed guard protection service for Sir Edward Heath, MP, Mr Tom King, MP, and other prominent members of state. But my new shift system, which I had intended to help me spend more time with my family, was to take a sudden twist.

Rebecca had celebrated her sixth birthday on 30 January and she was enjoying her school life. The legal team continued work on our claim of negligence and we had started to accumulate letters, reports, and other documents from our solicitor. We had both travelled to the Chambers at 1 Crown Office Row in London, the venue for meetings with our legal representatives and expert witnesses. These included David Hart, the barrister who would be responsible for representing and overseeing our case.

The team now consisted of two medical experts, a barrister, a solicitor and an occupational therapist, who would later become engaged in providing evidence regarding Chris's daily needs. She interviewed us at our home and compiled a report covering every aspect of Chris's disability. The opinions of the two medical investigators were now so strong that we had become confident of our case.

On 15 February, Chris attended the Royal Masonic Hospital in London where Mr Pat Soutter, an oncology specialist and one of our medical expert witnesses, examined her. He would provide an up to date report on her current prognosis.

Chris was always investigating the availability of new anti-cancer drugs and their release to the general public; her hopes and expectations were sometimes raised after discovering articles, often sensationalised, in the tabloids or on the television news. It was heartening to share her exhilaration when we heard about the discovery of a new medicine, but inevitably there was always the disillusionment that followed the hype, especially when The Department of Health announced that such-and-such a drug would not be available to the general public for another five years. Mr Soutter had knowledge of a new anti-cancer drug that was not readily available and he told Chris that he would make some enquires.

On 4 April, Chris and I had a four-hour meeting with the occupational therapist in our home. Her subsequent report detailed the plaintiff's disability needs, in accordance with the World Health Organisation's definitions and guidelines. A paragraph under the section explaining Chris's background information indicated her current condition and our present marital situation. In part, it reported that:

The strain of the past five years, the lack of counselling and practical support has seemingly destroyed their relationship.

It continued to explain that Chris would rather live alone with Rebecca and seek help from outsiders, than ask for my further support. It also confirmed that the ultimate destruction of a strong relationship and a happy marriage was caused by circumstances brought about by medical errors.

Soutter's prognosis following his examination of Chris was bleak and the information that he had about the new anti-cancer drug was disappointing. His report revealed that a slowly growing recurrence of Chris's cervical cancer would ultimately result in her death within the next year or so. Statistically, the predicted survival rate of five years for patients with progressive cervical cancer is fairly accurate. The drug he had enquired about Coumarin had not yet got a licence for marketing in Great Britain, nor indeed, anywhere else in the world. He was not, however, giving up hope completely, as he was still trying to get a special dispensation for Chris to take the drug. This would involve persuading the Hammersmith Hospital Drugs and Therapeutics Committee to prescribe it, providing Chris signed a disclaimer. She would have to wait for their decision.

It was clear that we had to make the best of whatever time we had left, especially while Chris's day-to-day health seemed reasonable. She had always wanted to take Rebecca on a special holiday to Disney World in Orlando, Florida. Ideally we would have preferred to wait a few years until she was ten which seemed a more sensible age for her to explore and enjoy the thrills and adventure of such a theme park but we arranged our trip for the second week of June, 1994. We chose early summer to avoid the overwhelming crowds and soaring high temperatures of peak season.

We explained to Rebecca that this was to be our holiday of a lifetime, a magical and exciting time and a dream that only came true for really well-behaved children whose parents had worked very hard to save their money for such a wonderful opportunity. Beneath the surface of excitement was the realism that this was probably going to be our last holiday together.

We took all the necessary steps to assure her that if Chris's health deteriorated while she was abroad, help would be at hand. She had to obtain a letter from her GP, confirming that she was fit to travel, a requirement of the tour operator for insurance purposes. It was also a safeguard in case she became ill and was in need of medical assistance, in which case her doctor could be contacted for advice. Its contents also explained the need for her to carry the vast array of medication on which she was so dependent. We had arranged a similar contingency plan four years earlier before travelling to Cyprus.

We both knew the American holiday was going to be expensive and I arranged a bank overdraft facility of £10,000 to cover the three-week break. Ordinarily, of course, we would have saved, as we had told Rebecca. This trip was not only a special treat for our daughter; but also it was also the fulfilment of a dream for Chris.

She had often talked about spending long relaxing days aboard an ocean liner on a Mediterranean cruise. I wanted to make that dream come true too, at least in part and persuaded her that we should include a short cruise in our American holiday. Of course, it was only short but we were thankful and overjoyed that Chris was well enough to spend seven days aboard a luxury liner. We would sail from Miami, visiting Jamaica, Mexico and the Cayman Islands.

Everything started well, except for an incident on the plane that caused some embarrassment. We were allocated the front seats on the aircraft to allow Chris easy access to the convenience. Naturally she would visit them more than most passengers, usually to empty her stoma bags. After each occasion she would spray the cubicle. Apparently this was not acceptable to some people. On the way back to her seat after her first visit, Chris passed an air hostess who was going to use the facility herself. However, the woman stopped just outside the lavatory and retreated to use another nearby. Minutes later she returned with her own container of air freshener and proceeded to spray the area, glaring back at Chris in the process. Exactly the same thing happened two or three more times during the flight.

Chris stopped me from approaching the air hostess, but I tried to explain that it was not the spraying that angered me, it was the woman's attitude and her unsympathetic approach to Chris's disability. The cabin crew knew of Chris's condition and she carried a card provided by the Stoma Association, indicating the necessity to use the facilities as a priority. I was sorry that I did not get the opportunity to say to her, "How would you like it if you had two stomas yourself?"

Despite this uneasy start, our holiday was everything that we had imagined. Our first week at the resort provided all the entertainment and enjoyment we had expected. Chris was able to walk short distances although she soon became exhausted, but a little later she was able to conserve her energy when we acquired the use of a wheelchair. I spent the first few days pushing her around, often with Rebecca sitting on her lap or standing on the footrest. Rebecca enjoyed being able to jump the queues for rides, because of the wheelchair. Her favourite was *It's A Small, Small World.* We all rode around it in a boat, Chris and Rebecca singing along with all the dolls from different nations.

We drove from Orlando to Miami to board our cruise ship. This was the only occasion on the holiday when Chris became unwell. It happened at the start of our cruise. We summoned the ship's doctor to our cabin and he was able to help control her acute abdominal pains, prescribing a stronger pain relief drug, to supplement her morphine supply. The cruise was wonderful. We had an exterior luxury cabin where Chris was able to relax on our private balcony enjoying the sea air. There was a crèche for Rebecca, which afforded Chris some real rest time. We visited the Cayman Islands, Jamaica and Mexico.

On our return home in July, Chris and Rebecca went to stay with her parents in Durham. She had planned to spend six weeks there during the school summer break and then return home to discuss our future. We were uncertain what to do for the best. It did not seem fair that Rebecca should miss the devotion and love of both of her parents. We shared the same feelings towards our daughter and it would have been extremely difficult for me to be away from her for any length of time. I also felt a strong sense of commitment and I knew in my heart that I could never leave them to fend for themselves. I had made this quite clear to Chris on many occasions.

As it turned out, we never had to make any clear-cut decisions. Chris decided to remain in Durham for a while. Her family was more than happy for the two of them to stay at their home and it was more beneficial for Chris in many ways. Naturally she had asked for my approval and of course I did not mind. It was what she wanted and it brought a certain respite for me.

TWENTY-TWO

Having an affair

Chris was now reliant on doctors in the northeast, most importantly for help in the management of the pain she suffered continually in her lower abdomen. In fairness to the decision she made to stay with her family, it was the best thing she could have done for herself and Rebecca. It was important to her to be near to her family, to people who could help and support her. She felt this particularly after hearing that there was nothing more that could be done. Had she returned home to Swindon and been successful in winning the compensation claim, her intention was to convert our home to make it more suitable for her disability so that her comfort and quality of life would be improved.

But the truth was that we were so uncertain. When our relationship was at its lowest at one point, we had even discussed selling our home, the intention being that Chris and Rebecca would live in a smaller house, with me living separately and relatively close by. That way we could still visit each other and share Rebecca. We simply did not know what would finally happen, though we knew that whatever we did, we would undoubtedly remain good friends.

Being on my own did not quite work out the way I had expected it to. I missed them both dreadfully and this was exacerbated when Rebecca cried during our telephone conversations, asking when I was coming to see her and Mummy. I promised her that I would come on my days off and eventually I committed myself to this routine, which continued for the remainder of their stay in Durham. I remembered telling Rebecca once that we were only three hundred miles from each other and that I could visit her and Mummy any time they needed me. Of course, the one-way journey could take up to six hours to drive. Quite often I would give Chris and her parents some time to themselves by taking Rebecca back home to

Swindon at weekends or during school breaks.

After a while they both got used to being at Chris's parents' home. As well as having the family to care for Chris there were also some nurses with whom she had trained at the nearby Dryburn Hospital who would occasionally visit. Some had qualified as district nurses and they would call to see her unofficially during their visits to other patients in the area. Their assistance was never too much trouble and they would regularly collect and deliver prescriptions to her home, organise and advise her on sanitary needs and recommend the latest disability aids. Chris looked forward to their company and talked openly with them about her illness. It was a way for her to release the pent-up stress and anxiety and finally to receive good counselling from people with whom she felt comfortable.

Knowing that there were friends around with a shared interest in Chris's past was a welcome boost to her morale and it gave her new hope to have people in the medical fraternity still caring about her. These contacts were replete with possibilities; maybe something more could still be done? Now that she had the opportunity to discuss the whole awful ordeal over again she gained renewed support from people who believed that they could help her increase her life expectancy. She found new faith in a future. Chris began to believe that she might yet survive.

Rebecca had joined the same primary school as her cousins. Her auntie lived nearby and provided the transport to take them all to school. She was content in her newfound surroundings. During the latter months of that year, Chris and her mother took Rebecca on weekend breaks to London, frequently accompanied by Chris's two sisters and their young daughters. They enjoyed many trips to theatres, flower shows and Chris's favourite annual event, The Ideal Home Exhibition at Earl's Court. These family trips were 'girls only' occasions; they provided many memorable moments for them all to cherish together. It was comforting for me to know that they were all very happy and making the most of each other's company. Most importantly, I was relieved that Chris had not become withdrawn, depressed, or dependent on everyone.

Meanwhile arguments continued back and forth between our legal representatives and the defendants' lawyers. Claims and counter-claims were now made by all parties responsible for the disgraceful catalogue of medical blunders. It had now reached the stage where each one of the defendants had issued a defence statement. These contained their own individual versions of events, justifying their mistakes. In short, they denied practically all of the allegations of negligence exposed by our medical experts. Instead of admitting liability now that the facts were clearly placed before them, they engaged in amateur and tedious manoeuvres that wasted time and, ultimately, public funds in the process. In effect these were cheap stalling tactics. Their motive for such obstructive behaviour was obvious. They knew that the plaintiff was a woman with a relatively short life expectancy. She would definitely cost them less in compensation if she died before the case was resolved.

In a report supplied by Professor Cotton on 27 August, 1994, in response to the defendants' defence statement, he concluded with this comment:

> *Finally, I remain confident that Christine Lucey has a very strong case, which can be supported by us as expert witnesses, and I think it is very unlikely that it will need to proceed to court.*

However, on 17 October, 1994, an application order was made before the Master Tennant in the London High Court, to set down a date for trial by judge, because neither of the defendants had provided any substantial evidence to dismiss the numerous claims of negligence brought against them. Nor did they admit liability; at one point the solicitors acting for the second defendants had made a contemptible and insulting effort to circumvent the evidence by offering one hundred and fifty thousand pounds, without admitting liability or prejudice.

The High Court order would allow each party to prepare for

the trial, which would be set six months from the date of application. The rules allowed each side to produce up to three expert medical and three non-medical witnesses. We had already utilised our witnesses months before and had provided their completed reports. Now the defendants had no choice but to stop their stalling tactics and start to abide by the rules of the High Court. The Master Tennant, who acted as a kind of referee, had stipulated a strict timetable in respect of exchanging statements, medical reports and other relevant information, providing a formula for all the legal representatives to adhere. Hopefully, this would ensure a speedy trial.

On November 25, arrangements were being made by the defendants' medical expert to examine Chris, with a view to supplying their own prognosis report. She was to attend the Royal Marsden Hospital in London some time the following month. They were also to make arrangements for a rehabilitation costs consultant and an architect to prepare opposing reports to ours; these would either agree with or undermine our witnesses' information concerning modification of our home to meet Chris's daily needs.

While all this was happening, Chris decided that I was having an affair. It was the only reason she could attribute to my sudden change in attire. I had started to wear a round-neck jumper. It was three days before Christmas, my Mum had arrived and was staying for the holidays and I had brought Chris and Rebecca back home for the festive season. My sister had bought me a Marks and Spencer jumper a few days before, an early Christmas present. I wasn't too keen on the pattern, and normally loathed wearing anything that covered my neck, preferring V-neck tops.

The suspicions began when we were sitting in the lounge. I had just finished getting ready to go out for a drink with my friend, Alan. Chris was moody and short-tempered. The long journey from Durham the previous day had left her tired and irritable. Maybe it had also something to do with the medication she was taking, which often left her feeling drowsy and affected her personality, a change that I had noticed during the last months. Perhaps she was cross that I seemed to be enjoying my new bachelor status, free from the responsibility of caring for her and Rebecca. Not that it was quite like that. Most of my time had been taken up with work commitment or visiting them in Durham.

I had never actually been interested in meeting another woman, at least not in the sense of having a relationship. It was not ethical. I was still married and my wife was dying. I also had Rebecca's welfare to consider. Under the circumstances, however, Chris's jealousy and suspicions were understandable.

Before I left to go out that evening she started to argue with me, saying in front of everyone that she could not care less if I was seeing someone else, she did not give a damn what I was doing. She was going back to Durham in the New Year and I could please myself because she did not need me any more.

I told her not to be so stupid. Rebecca immediately defended her. She said, "Don't call Mummy stupid, you're the one who's stupid, Daddy." Then she cuddled up to Chris. I felt hurt and rejected but I realised that Rebecca had simply seen me as the cause for upsetting Mummy. Naturally she wanted to protect her from my abrupt comments. Thankfully children are very resilient and do not bear grudges

Though I do not think Chris was convinced that I was not seeing somebody else, mercifully, the incident was soon forgotten and we had a pleasant time for the remainder of their stay.

They returned to Durham on 4 January, 1995. I continued the ritual of visiting on my days off, but there were no further remarks about my social life. We each continued our separate lives.

During the first few weeks of January there was very little communication involving our negligence case. The solicitors acting on behalf of the second defendants were still delaying and had not even made contact about the medical prognosis examination that should have taken place in December. Chris was not prepared to travel all the way to London at this stage just for a second opinion on her life expectancy for their benefit; Mr Pat Soutter's prognosis report should have sufficed.

Meanwhile she had more important issues to consider. Her quality of life was declining. She was now attending three major hospitals in Durham, Sunderland and Newcastle, in a vain and desperate attempt to find a specialist who could help control her agonising abdominal pain. She was eventually successful in finding an oncologist consultant who was able to administer suitable drugs. But in February Chris's health deteriorated further. Once again she was being admitted to hospital regularly for blood transfusions. Her vaginal bleeding had worsened and she was now unable to leave her parents' home except to go to hospital.

She would spend most of the day lying on the settee, her knees raised to ease the pain. Her legs would shake uncontrollably, even when she was asleep. The movements were similar to the withdrawal symptoms that a drug addict experiences. She was unable to hold a conversation without lapsing into semi-consciousness, waking a few moments later to continue on the same subject. She had become dependent on a visit from the district nurse every day to help her take her medication, to bathe and to change her incontinence pads. Her body image had further deteriorated; she was still reliant on steroids, she was distended and relied on the use of a walking stick on the rare occasions when she moved from one room to the next.

I offered to take a few weeks off work to spend time with Chris and Rebecca, but Chris now refused my help. She didn't want me to waste my annual leave, suggesting I should save it for later in the year when I could take them both somewhere special. I wanted to be with her, but she was right: there was nothing that I could do that everyone else was capable of doing. I respected her decision and said I would come up if she needed me. She continued to have both good and bad days over the following two months.

At last there was a breakthrough from the defendants' solicitors. Chris had received a phone call from Mr John Czul, our solicitor and she managed to telephone me soon afterwards to tell me the good news. The Ministry of Defence had admitted liability. There was no dispute and they would compensate her in full! She was so pleased that they had admitted their mistake; it seemed to prove without a shadow of doubt that there was gross negligence both on their part and on that of the co-defendants. However, the Ministry had accepted full responsibility, which meant that the Swindon Health Authority was absolved from all allegations of negligence pertaining to the misreporting of smear tests. In effect, they had got off lightly, to say the least.

Just at the eleventh hour Chris had always seemed to find something new to help her fight on a little further, despite her ailing condition. Now she would never have to give up. She could go ahead and try to secure the future she wanted for Rebecca and her parents. Everything seemed much more within her reach. She did not have to worry about either coming back to Swindon or moving to a smaller home. Now we could sell our house, pay off the mortgage and divide the proceeds.

On 10 March, 1995, Mr Czul sent a letter to Chris confirming that the Ministry of Defence had conceded liability. There seemed no reason whatsoever for the case to be tried in the High Court.

Chris had previously mentioned buying a small bungalow close to her family, which made sense. It would eliminate the need for her to negotiate the stairs in her parents' home. Her parents could then move from their semi-detached council house and into the bungalow with Chris and Rebecca. She said that when she died Rebecca would return home to live with me but her Mum and Dad could have the bungalow as a gift. In return they would eventually bequeath their estate to the grandchildren, including Rebecca.

At the end of March, the Treasury solicitor forwarded an interim payment to Chris of fifteen thousand pounds. Negotiations were taking place for further funds to be made available to enable her to buy the bungalow as a matter of urgency. In retrospect, it can be seen that the defendants were, by this time, being extremely co-operative. The bungalow cost sixty-nine thousand pounds. There was more than enough to cover the purchase price as they had already made an original offer of one hundred and fifty thousand pounds, even before admitting liability.

The final settlement, however, could now be as high as three or four hundred thousand pounds. It would be calculated from a special damages report. This included loss of income for both of us, a personal injury claim, capital expenditure and other calculations. Whatever the outcome of the settlement, it could never compensate for the distress and suffering Chris had been through or the fact that the carelessness of those responsible had destroyed our lives.

Chris never got the opportunity to buy the bungalow. Her parents and family would later contest the issue and begin a dispute over the legalities behind the potential purchase of the property. Their dissatisfaction and selfishness was revealed on the one day of all days that should have been free of all selfish thoughts. It left me stunned and shaken in disbelief.

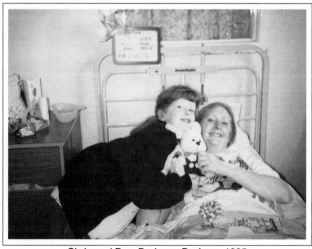

Chris and Rex, Dryburn, Durham, 1995

Twenty-Three

The Rose

On Monday, April 24, Chris was taken into Dryburn Hospital. I received a phone call from her father, who told me she had haemorrhaged again and had to have further blood transfusions. He suggested that I should come up to Durham as her condition had become very serious and he did not think she would pull through this time. I travelled up that evening.

Chris was alone in a side ward, too ill to be with other patients. The familiar array of drip pumps was around her bedside; three units of blood had been given during the day. She lay asleep with her legs bent in the position she had become accustomed to for so long, her knees trembling as usual. I sat next to her and waited for her to wake up, but she continued to sleep. Eventually I left the ward, leaving her in this unconscious state and drove to her parents' home.

Rebecca was asleep when I walked into her bedroom. I picked up Lulu, her teddy bear, from the floor and placed it beside her. We had bought Lulu for her when she was two years old. It was her favourite; she took it everywhere. I kissed her on the cheek and whispered, "Goodnight, darling. Mummy and Daddy love you so much."

The next day I collected Rebecca from school and took her to see her mother. Chris was awake. Rebecca lay on the bed beside her and they hugged each other, murmuring a few words. Chris had asked me to bring in a legal form from our solicitor, which she would sign, giving me power of attorney to act on her behalf in signing any legal document. She still wanted to proceed with the purchase of the bungalow. As she slowly signed, I looked and saw that she had misspelled her surname: *C Llucey*. Other members of her family then arrived and, as we were leaving, she managed a faint wave to Rebecca before closing her eyes. She fell asleep, totally unaware of her other visitors.

I took a single red rose to her on Wednesday morning and placed it in a vase with some other flowers. I had bought it earlier from a street trader, an old woman, selling individual flowers in the market place in Durham.

Chris was asleep. I waited a moment and then left without disturbing her. I returned that evening and was sitting near her bed when she awoke. I had the opportunity to talk to her for a short while. Chris looked at me and said, "This is it, this time, Don, isn't it?" I held her hand as I had done before and said she would be fine. She smiled weakly. "I've been a right bitch, haven't I?" she whispered.

"No you haven't. What made you say that?"

"Because I came here to Durham and left you on your own".

I told her she'd had no choice, They'd given up on her in the south, yet she was able to have further treatment in the north. And she'd had the opportunity to spend some quality time with her family. I squeezed her frail hand and said, "I still love you, Chris."

She gazed at me, still with that faint smile on her face, and said, "Do you? Do you really?"

"Yes, darling," I replied, then, as she slowly closed her eyes, she murmured, "I'm so pleased, Don. Now I can die in peace."

On Friday, 28 April, Rebecca saw her Mum for the last time. They still managed their hug as they lay huddled close to each other and as we left her that evening, Chris said her final words to her: "Goodbye, darling. I love you".

During the weekend the doctors continued to administer blood transfusions. She had haemorrhaged several times over the course of a few days. At twelve-thirty on Monday afternoon, 1 May, I arrived at the hospital, having received a phone call to say that the doctor responsible for her care had made a decision to stop any further blood transfusions. There was no other course of action for them to take; Chris was losing blood as quickly as it was being administered. During the weekend, they had tried everything possible, to no avail. The lifeline that had kept her alive for the past week was now humanely terminated. She was left to die.

Her parents sat near her, drinking tea from the hospital's best bone china tea set, their faces showing no signs of emotion, as Chris stared into oblivion. I squeezed past them, taking a linen handkerchief from my pocket, weeping as I leant forward to kiss her for the final time. Tiny beads of perspiration rolled down her face. I gently wiped the moisture from her forehead and then the tears from my eyes. I whispered, "Goodbye, my darling Chris. I still love you", and slipped quietly out of the room into an adjacent side ward to be alone with my thoughts.

The rest of her family arrived and hustled in to see her. This time the decision to allow her the privacy to die alone was not mine to make. Eight members of her family had gathered around her bed. The door to her room was slightly ajar and I could hear them discussing her past and the suffering she had endured. They talked of camping holidays when they were younger and about the bungalow. They were drinking tea and eating digestive biscuits. Some were laughing about the good old days they had all shared. Chris remained in the same lifeless position, her eyes gazing upwards as she waited for her life to end.

I wondered if they knew that a person's hearing is the last of the senses to fade from a dying body. Chris could probably hear every word they were saying and would have to endure their drone for quite a while longer before her last breath allowed her the peace she so greatly deserved.

It was three o'clock that afternoon and my thoughts were with Rebecca as I hurried along the corridor on my way out to collect her from school. I stopped briefly to talk to the Macmillan nurse in her office. She was one of the members of staff responsible for ensuring that Chris passed away peacefully and without pain. I had watched earlier as another nurse injected a dose of morphine into her thigh. Chris flinched and groaned slightly as the syringe entered her skin, her only movement and sound as she lay unconscious. The nurse had reassured the onlookers that she was in no pain.

I now wanted some indication, without sounding morbid, of the length of time Chris had before she died. I knew it would take me an hour to drive Rebecca to her cousin's home and then return; I was not bringing Rebecca to see Chris, no matter what anyone else thought. The nurse was sympathetic and understood my question; it was a normal thing to ask. She was trained in caring for the terminally ill, had probably witnessed a lot of deaths and specialised in bereavement counselling.

Rebecca ran across the playground shouting, "Daddy, Daddy, take me in to see Mummy. I haven't seen her for days."

"Not today, darling," I replied as she leapt into my arms. "She's not very well. Maybe tomorrow." I couldn't say anything else. I had to lie. She knew Mummy was ill and had gone into hospital to get better. It had always been like that, ever since she was a year old.

I recalled the many times Rebecca had told her Mummy that she wanted to be a doctor so that when she grew up she could help her to get better. She would not get that opportunity. I held back my emotions as I realised that by this time tomorrow Mummy would have died. I held her tightly in my arms once more before I left her at her cousins' house. As she scampered off to play with them, she called back over her shoulder, "Give my love to Mummy, Daddy. By-ee…" The tears flooded my eyes as I drove back to the hospital.

The distressing hours of waiting continued. It was ten o'clock that evening and 'The Woman Who Wouldn't Die' was still holding on; she would not give up. The nursing staff had moved her over onto her side and she seemed more peaceful and comfortable like that, as though she were simply asleep. I wished they had done it ten hours earlier. I walked past the side ward, where there was a small window with an opening in the curtains and I risked a glance. The same relatives filled the room. They had been sitting there practically all day. I returned to the adjacent side ward, a self-imposed exile, away from Chris's family. I had felt unwelcome from the moment I arrived, inept and out of place. Whenever I had peeked in to see my wife, my presence was ignored.

At one o'clock in the morning I was sitting waiting like everyone else, when a priest pushed open the door. He apologised, saying, "I'm looking for a lady who is very ill… dying… I think I've got the wrong room, haven't I?" I scowled at him, then stood up and pointed to the room opposite. "The lady you're looking for is my wife. She's in that room there." He stammered an apology as he closed the door behind him. Chris's family had done their duty and summoned the priest for the last rites. I could not help being brusque. I felt hot and irritable. Someone had to suffer. This time it was the priest. I decided to go outside for some fresh air and sat in my car for a while. It was two o'clock, Chris was still alive.

I must have fallen asleep for a while. I looked at my watch: it was now three o'clock. I felt calm and more relaxed. It was so quiet. I went back inside and walked down the corridor towards the side ward. A nurse came out of the staff room and walked towards me. She told me that everyone had gone and Chris had passed away. I pushed the door open to the side ward and she walked in behind me. "Now you can have as much time as you want with her, Don, you're both finally alone. She's at peace now and will be pleased you're here". The nurse's words summed up the long, lingering journey Chris had taken to her final resting place. Now the fight was over. She would suffer no more.

Chris lay still beneath a clean white linen sheet. Her body was perfectly straight, no more bent and trembling knees. Her hair was brushed back neat and tidy, her eyes were closed and she looked at peace. Now there was no more pain for her to worry about. The windows were open, the curtains moved gently with the early morning breeze that flowed softly into the room. The only noise to be heard was the birds singing their dawn chorus. The room was free from the derangement of chairs, trays of empty crockery, and medical paraphernalia. The single red rose that I had brought for her days before stood alone on the window sill, as though she had commanded it to be left there. I walked over and gently touched her face with my fingertips: her skin was cool and soft. I whispered, "Sleep, my darling Christine. You have suffered enough".

I knelt down beside her bed and prayed, asking God to look after His child. I asked His forgiveness for the time I was angry and shouted, mistakenly blaming him for her illness when I had first been told she had cancer and was going to die. I stood up and walked back to the window; looked out at the trees. The birds had stopped singing, as if they had sensed the need for silence. A small mark of respect.

I cast my mind back over the six years my wife had struggled to stay alive and I cried as I thought of the last time Rebecca and Chris lay close to each other a few days earlier, now separated in this life, forever. I left the room and whispered my last words to her: "Goodbye, my darling Chris... we'll miss you".

I went into the ward sister's office and collected Chris's personal belongings. I thanked the staff for all their help. As I walked out of the hospital for the final time, I remembered how Chris had spoken about her fond memories of Dryburn Hospital. This was where she had trained as a young nurse before joining the Queen Alexandra's Royal Army Nursing Corp, almost twenty years earlier.

Now it was finally over, I had to think of my own mental well-being and that of my daughter. It was my responsibility to ensure that Rebecca was allowed slowly to adjust to and accept the loss of a mother and friend. I would supervise that process, with all the care and patience it took, no matter what I had to sacrifice.

TWENTY-FOUR

Mummy died this morning

A few hours later, the family congregated at Chris's parents' home. Her mother stood ironing clothes, while her father watched breakfast television. They talked of the difficulties they had experienced in looking after their sick daughter during the past nine months and how much everyone else had had to help. There were still no tears nor the slightest indication that they were in mourning. I thought that perhaps their grief was on hold, this composure a way of showing their relief that Chris was no longer suffering. Perhaps it was a demonstration of how strong they still were.

The subject of purchasing the bungalow was mentioned and I said that I would have to talk to Mr Czul, our solicitor, about the current position. It made me wonder if that was their main consideration.

I knew it was time to tell Rebecca. I called her in from the garden, where she was playing with her cousins and took her for a drive. We ended up in a small village nearby called Meadowfield. I felt as though some mysterious force had guided me there as I parked outside the very church where Chris and I had been married. I had not been to sleep all night. I was very tired. I did not want to tell Rebecca that her Mum had died. But I knew that I had to tell her sooner or later, before someone else did.

We sat outside on the newly mowed lawn and Rebecca huddled up close to me, her curiosity and impatience starting to show. I tried to hold back my tears, but I couldn't. "What's wrong, Daddy?" she asked. I began by telling her that this was the church in which Mummy and Daddy were married and I wanted to sit outside this very special place with her because it was what Mummy would have wanted us to do. I talked briefly about Mummy's illness and explained the reasons why she had to go into hospital. Then I said, "You know Mummy was very ill last week."

"Yes, Daddy, I know," she said, in a matter-of-fact way, looking at me as if she were still waiting to be told something new.

"Well, darling, Mummy was *very* ill and…" The tears streamed down my face as I tried to say what had happened.

"What, Daddy? What's happened?" Rebecca too began to cry. She had sensed something was awfully wrong.

"Darling," I said, "Mummy died this morning and she's gone to heaven".

Rebecca stared at me in disbelief for a split second then screamed in utter anguish. She cried and cried, shouting, "Why didn't you take me to see her, why didn't you take me to see her, Daddy?" hitting my chest with her tiny fists, again and again and again.

"I couldn't, darling, I couldn't. Mummy was too ill," I sobbed.

My lovely daughter wrapped her arms around me, both of us now overcome with grief, and she said, "I'll never be happy again, Daddy."

We hugged each other tightly, both crying hard, not caring about the world. Finally, I pulled my handkerchief from my pocket and she wiped the tears from her eyes. She handed it to me and I did the same and then gave it back to her. I told her it was the same handkerchief that I had used to wipe Mummy's tears from her eyes. Now it was a very special handkerchief that she could keep forever.

Suddenly a small dog appeared from nowhere, jumping in between us and interrupting our moment of grief. It ran off and then came back again, barking playfully and nudging Rebecca. She started to giggle and called out, "Come here, boy. Come here". It started to lick her face, prompting more giggles, and eventually returned to its master. The dog's arrival had signalled an appropriate time to end our discussion. We moved on to sit on some swings in a nearby park, kicking our feet forward and back in a rocking motion, both of us talking to Mummy in heaven as we stared up to the sky. After a few hours of reminiscing, discreet shouting to rid the anger from our thoughts and a fair bit of crying, we returned to the house to pack Rebecca's clothes and to say goodbye to her cousins and grandparents. We had decided to go back home to Swindon.

Rebecca was still crying, clutching the handkerchief tightly in her hands, as we left to drive back that evening. Earlier I had organised the funeral arrangements and had registered the death. Chris was to be buried on Friday, 5 May.

On Wednesday morning Rebecca gave me the handkerchief and asked if we could put it somewhere safe. I placed it inside a small purse that had belonged to Chris and then inside a cabinet with other family mementoes.

On Thursday Rebecca returned to the same junior school that she had attended before going away to Durham. It was important for her to continue socialising with other children and to get back to her schooling as quickly as possible to help her to adjust and cope with the bereavement. We discussed what she wanted to do and I gave her the option of going to Mummy's funeral or staying with a friend. She decided to stay with her friend that evening.

*

On Friday the funeral took place in Durham. The church was filled with friends and relatives. The coffin lay at the front near the altar. I sat staring at it and looking at the empty seat next to me that had been reserved for Rebecca. Chris would have understood her decision to stay at home.

Later, I threw a handful of soil onto the coffin and placed two wreaths near the grave. One was from me, the other, in the shape of a teddy bear, from Rebecca. On the card she had written the words: *To Little Mummy, love, Rebecca, xxx.*

She had called Chris 'Little Mummy' from an early age, using it as an affectionate term for the first time when she was about three. It's likely that Rebecca can remember more events from that period of happy reunion than from any other time. Mother and daughter had missed each other for so long and then had fourteen whole months of hugs and kisses to enjoy. They had played together on the carpet, building things with Lego blocks and they had watched *Neighbours* together, Rebecca jumping up and down singing 'Nay-nors, Nay-nors' every time she heard the signature tune. I remember feeling slightly rejected back then. After all, I had had to look after our daughter practically on my own throughout those fourteen months.

Jean had been a supportive help but she was only part time. I cared for Rebecca in the evenings, at night and early mornings. She was my little girl and we had so much fun together, as well as the naughty times, of course, when she used to throw tantrums and I would tap her leg gently to show her who was in charge. I remember her crying and asking for her 'Little Mummy' Then she would say, "Dada, when is Little Mummy coming home?" I would hug her and tell her, "Soon, baby, soon." That 'soon' had taken such a long time for both of us. Now she would not see her 'Little Mummy' ever again.

At the end of the service the mourners mingled, hugging and shaking hands, expressing their condolences. Some were weeping. I moved towards my family and friends to thank them for attending, then towards Christine's relatives. Several members of her family ignored my attempt to express my sympathy to them: they completely shunned my gestures of consolation. Naturally I was shocked and distressed by their actions and I could not understand how they could be so cold and inconsiderate, especially on such a sad day. I asked other relatives what was wrong, what could I possibly have done to deserve such heinous and insulting behaviour. No one seemed to know, but it was suggested that they were simply overcome with grief.

The funeral procession left the cemetery and returned to the family residence; friends and relatives gathered once more to offer their condolences. My isolation continued; though some members of my family and some of Christine's relatives and friends gave me their support and encouragement. This helped me to endure my feelings about being shunned at the cemetery.

Before I left Durham to return home that day, I approached my father-in-law, hoping to get an explanation for this unbelievable display of acrimony. His explanation was vague. He told me not to worry because they were stricken with grief and had probably not realised their insensitivity.

On my way home, I tried to analyse the situation. I turned it over and over in my mind, but I just could not understand it. Later that evening a phone call was to give me an indication and a sickening clue, though I would never know the whole of the reason. Even to this day, there are certain members of Chris's family that I have not seen or even talked to since the funeral. Surprisingly, those with whom I did keep in contact would not discuss the matter.

*

When I called at her friend's house, Rebecca wanted to stay another night with Emily and asked if I would collect her on Saturday morning. I told her that Mummy's funeral was lovely and her teddy bear wreath had been left alongside mine. I promised to take her to see the grave when the headstone was erected. It had been only three days since Chris died but Rebecca was incredibly resilient and was happy staying with her friend. Their minds were preoccupied with joyful, innocent, childish things. I knew that there would be plenty of time later for crying: time for both of us. We embraced and I went to visit my family for the evening. I sat talking with my Mum and sister. They liked Chris and would miss her tremendously. We had many memories to reminisce. They invited me to stay overnight. They knew I would be on my own and as usual they fussed about my welfare.

At nine o'clock that evening I received a call on my mobile

phone from Chris's brother. He said he had been asked to contact me on behalf of his parents. The conversation that followed caused me to feel extremely uncomfortable and aroused my suspicions regarding the earlier events at the funeral.

Chris's parents wanted to know what was happening about the bungalow and were wondering if they were still going to receive it. I told my brother-in-law that I did not know and asked how they could even be thinking about this on the day that their daughter was buried. He said that he knew it was not a good time to phone, but they wanted to know. He referred to other members of the family who had expressed their concern. They thought that it was right that the parents should be given the Bungalow because Chris had promised she would buy the property for her parents. I repeated that I simply did not know what was happening and would have to contact the solicitor on Monday. I told him that if it was something that Christine had promised, there should not be any problem. He continued by saying that everyone thought I should already have the answer because I had Chris's power of attorney. I told him this was true but it had only been done to allow me to sign on Chris's behalf when contracts were exchanged. It had not reached that stage and I was not sure of the present situation. I said I would also ask my solicitor to contact them directly. "Make sure you do then," he concluded, "'bye."

I couldn't believe what I had just heard. All they could think about was whether or not they were still entitled to own the bungalow. My mother and sister were disgusted at the thought of Chris's family enquiring about money, only hours after her funeral. I wondered if this was the reason for the animosity that I had experienced in Durham. Did they know something of which I was not aware? Maybe they had already talked to Mr Czul, our solicitor. Perhaps he had told them it depended on me or on the contents of the will. I didn't know and quite frankly, I really didn't care.

It could wait until Monday.

TWENTY-FIVE

Settlement

Rebecca and I returned home that weekend and began our lives without Chris. Both of us kept occupied as much as we could. We cried often. In some small way this helped us to cope with the fact that we would never see Chris again. There was a strange atmosphere in the house, a feeling of emptiness in every room. The hardest task was packing up items of clothing and other personal effects that had belonged to Chris. It was going to take us both a long time to come to terms with the loss of a mother and a wife. I let Rebecca sleep in my bed for a while to give her comfort and a feeling of security. Before she went to sleep each night she would cry for her Mummy.

On Monday I contacted our solicitor and related the telephone call that I had received from Chris's family. I mentioned their concern about the purchase of the bungalow and their view that they were still entitled to it. He confirmed that I had relinquished my responsibility as power of attorney for Chris when she passed away. Now there was no possibility of their having the ownership of the bungalow. If Chris had lived and the purchase had materialised, then it would have been a different story. He said that he would contact them and explain the situation.

I felt that the family had already blamed me for stopping Chris's parents from owning the bungalow and that this was the reason for their display of unforgivable behaviour at her funeral. I could not think of any other excuse. Surely if they needed something so badly all they had to do was ask? I would probably have bought the bungalow for them, irrespective of the amount of the final compensation. The repercussions were to continue for a long time, despite the fact that Chris's family would eventually receive a substantial sum for their part in caring for her during those final nine months of her life.

The rules began to change as soon as the defendants heard that Chris had died. Notwithstanding their admission in a letter two months earlier to our solicitor, "confirming liability and not wanting to withstand a long fight in the courts", they now began to ask for further documented evidence to support the compensation claim. With Chris now out of the equation, the original costs prepared by our rehabilitation consultant were now redundant. They asked for a fresh report.

Our solicitor had to employ another agency to produce the complex details that would include numerous calculations relevant to claims for Rebecca and me. The defendants demanded yet more evidence; they now challenged existing facts. Now these faceless bureaucrats could take as long as they wanted; they seemed determined to drag their heels even more than before. We waited: my faith in justice and my determination to win for Chris and Rebecca would not falter and Mr Czul and his team of experts would patiently provide any information that was requested.

After six weeks I returned to work; Nanny Jean was once again looking after Rebecca on a part-time basis. The months soon passed. After Rebecca's school holidays I decided to employ a full-time nanny while I was at work. But in the end this didn't happen quite as I wanted. After several weeks and the experience of three very short-term 'employed' nannies, I decided to take a career break and look after my daughter myself. She was unhappy and cried incessantly. She missed her mother so much. The words that Rebecca had blurted out when I told her Chris had died and gone to heaven still haunted me: "I'll never be happy again, Daddy". I was very concerned for her welfare.

I knew that Rebecca would cope better with me looking after her rather than someone else. It worked: she began to settle better at school. She started horse riding, and later in the year she went to a private school. This was something Chris had always wanted for her and it was my way of fulfilling another of Chris's dreams. Rebecca became happier; her young life could progress. Her memories of her mother's suffering would gradually fade, but she would never forget the love they had shared. She would always know that Mum was still there, watching over and protecting her.

*

In September, 1997, I resigned from the Wiltshire Constabulary. Rebecca and I slowly adapted to the changes in our lives, as most single parents with children do. I had one brief relationship that really constituted little more than companionship for Rebecca and me. I never found anyone that was really compatible. I was never interested in looking for someone to replace Chris; the circumstances of her illness had changed our whole lives but not our real love for each other. She was an amazing woman, kind and generous, with an enormous consideration and compassion for others. Chris was very gregarious and greatly enjoyed socialising. We had been married for sixteen years and had shared so many happy times together, the proudest and most rewarding moment being the birth of our daughter. Rebecca was everything to me now and I would ensure that she continued to lead a full and happy life until the day she finds a partner to love and care for her.

Meeting after meeting took place with our legal representatives and expert witnesses. Now that Chris had died, our compensation claim was in abeyance or as Mr Czul put it, 'in limbo'. He would now have to abide by the stiff rules of the legal system and go through the long-winded procedure of obtaining Grants of Probate and Representation from the High Court, in order to allow three Executors, myself, Mr Czul, and a member of Chris's family, to represent Chris as former plaintiffs and to act in accordance within the law relating to conditions set out in her will.

It had turned into a whole new ball game, with Rebecca and I as plaintiffs, included in the Estate of Christine Lucey. It was a major setback. Legal Aid was suspended and a new application had to be made on behalf of Rebecca. Six months after Chris's death, the court finally granted permission for proceedings to continue and Rebecca was allowed legal aid. The delay had allowed the defendants an opportunity to sit back, while we made all the running. In real terms, three years of our hard work was now practically wasted, but the medical experts' evidence stood fast. Nothing could change the substantive facts stacked against the defendants, no matter what they said now.

Three years were to pass before our solicitor and his team of experts finally put a stop to the defendant's games of brinkmanship over the medical evidence. The time had come for them to appear before a High Court judge. Our barrister, David Hart, was ready to challenge their barrister, Ian Burnett; each referring to the bundles of evidence they had accumulated over six years.

On Tuesday, 24 March, 1998, I walked into the High Court in London, ready to appear as a witness and give evidence. I was prepared to face the barrister representing The Ministry of Defence. I knew that the four-day trial would be gruelling but I believed that we had the chance to win and walk away not only with compensation, but also with the satisfaction of having exposed the people responsible for the death of Christine Lucey, a loving mother and wife. I really wanted to expose every detail of their medical blunders and through the eyes of the media, to warn every one who has ever blindly trusted doctors that they can and do make catastrophic mistakes.

But Mr Czul and the expert witnesses were waiting for me inside the main door with some news. An offer had been put forward by the defendants' counsel. Mr Czul had been right: he had predicted that they would try for an out-of-court settlement but I was not tempted. I rejected the offer. Their offer was twenty percent less than the total quantum figure but our barrister said that it was a good offer and that I should take it. I turned to Mr Czul and to the rehabilitation expert, Ms Verne Ann Convey. They showed me some newspaper articles that depicted compensation claims and the meagre awards some unfortunate victims had received. They urged me to accept the offer, as they were apprehensive that the judge, as he had done in other cases, would slice chunks out of the figures that were calculated in the Special Damages Report. Its contents included not only a general damages claim, but also a loss of dependency claim, that is, the services of wife and mother, the value of care and other expenditure in respect of Durham, the claim by Chris's parents for their role in caring for their daughter.

Though my motive for wanting to fight was not greed, my confidence had gone. Adrenalin was coursing through my body. I was alone; the choice was mine to make. Our team was still prepared to continue with a trial, but it was up to me.

After a few hours of deliberation, the defendants made a new offer increasing their original figure. I thought of Rebecca and the gamble of a four-day trial. Was I prepared to take the risk of losing compensation that would ultimately provide a secure financial future for her? I felt that I had no choice but to accept and both parties then appeared before the High Court judge to inform him that the matter had been resolved. A settlement had been reached.

TWENTY-SIX

I have read the papers in this case and, as a hard-bitten judge of many years experience I could not fail to be moved by the suffering of Mrs Lucey

Mr Justice Alliott expressed his learned opinion. Mr Ian Burnett, counsel for the defendants, expressed his regret on behalf of The Ministry of Defence and stated that he was pleased that the settlement had been reached without the need for Mr Lucey to go through the harrowing experience of giving evidence to the court. He expressed his best wishes to Rebecca and to me for the future.

Our barrister, David Hart, made reference to the judge about my role in looking after Rebecca: "He stepped into the breach to look after Rebecca and has continued to do so," he said. As we walked from Court Thirteen, I stopped and looked back along the corridor. I watched the defendants' counsel hurrying out of the building and vowed there and then to tell the story that would describe how their clients had contributed to ending the life of a brave young woman who had paid the ultimate price for trusting doctors.

Mr Czul was pleased; his job was done. Now he could close the file on the Lucey Case forever. The barrister and two of our expert witnesses, Mr Pat Soutter MD, and Ms Verne Ann Convey shook my hand and congratulated me on the settlement.

I walked along the corridor with Mr Czul and his assistant and into the Great Hall. I was struck by the splendour of the magnificent nineteenth-century architecture. The mosaic floor in the main hall stretched its entire length, two hundred and thirty feet from north to south. The elaborately carved oak-panelled walls and ceilings were also magnificent. Intricately designed archways spanned the eighty-two foot high building. A stone column hung several feet from the floor; it had been deliberately left unfinished by the architect, George Street, apparently intended as a mark of respect, since he believed that only Jesus Christ Himself could create a perfect building. An oil painting portrayed a scene of Queen Victoria opening the Royal Courts in 1882. Statues of loyal subjects, lords, judges and chancellors, were featured throughout the majestic building.

What a contrast all this splendour was to the dull and uninviting surroundings of Court Thirteen only minutes earlier. Judge Alliott's sympathetic and moving tribute resounded in my head as we walked towards the exit. His comments exemplified my mixed feelings of despair combined with admiration for Chris. Mr Czul stopped by a large display cabinet containing various costumes and wigs worn by judges, past and present. He turned towards me, shook my hand and said, "That's it, Don, it's all over!"

"Yes," I said, "it is John. Thanks for everything you've done. It's been a long struggle, hasn't it?"

"Yes," he replied, "you're right, it certainly has."

His paralegal assistant, Mr Gurbir, followed behind, carrying large bundles of court documents and files, as we continued past the enquiry desk. Lawyers and plaintiffs mingled with barristers dressed in black gowns with white, tightly curled wigs. Security staff searched visitors coming in and scanned their bodies with hand-held metal detectors. A statue of George Street stood nearby, eerily watching over his creation. We walked through the double porch, its upper arch adorned with meticulously carved wooden statues of eminent judges and lawyers. We passed through the large metal gates onto The Strand and the busy streets of London.

There were no raised hands or jubilant cries of victory. We were not swamped by hordes of camera-crews, press photographers or reporters on the pavements outside, often the scene following successful claims outside the country's most influential law courts. I did not feel victorious or jubilant after being awarded the personal injury claim of almost half a million pounds. I felt flat. I had not won real justice for Chris in the way that I had expected. I felt guilty that I had not seized my opportunity to expose the catalogue of medical mistakes in public. I had wanted to shame The National Health Service and the Ministry of Defence but instead I had accepted an offer. It was a pay-off. And my conscience was bothering me.

Mr Czul and his assistant paused before stepping into the taxi and looked up at the tall spires towering above the historic building. I was unable to share their enthusiasm for a job well done as the taxi drove us away from the Royal Courts of Justice. I looked pensively out of the window as they continued to gaze at the prestigious landmark. Mr Czul launched into his guided tour routine like a novice courier, showing local cab drivers the sights of London. Mr Gurbir broke into his commentary and said, "We didn't need the files or the video tape after all, John."

"No, we didn't, Gurbir," I said, cutting his conversation short before Mr Czul had the chance to answer. I wasn't listening properly to what was said after that, thinking instead of a comment Chris had made on the recording: "I hope this tape will be of some use for those who are interested in our case."

I apologised for my brusqueness and said, "You're right, Gurbir, we didn't need the tape or anything in the end."

He nodded his head sympathetically and said, "It's okay, Don, I understand."

I had been in the solicitor's office the day before, when we watched the recording to check the viewing quality. Mr Gurbir wanted to make sure it wasn't damaged in any way. I remembered him checking and double-checking with London court officials, to ensure they had a television and video player available to allow the judge to watch the tape.

Mr Gurbir was the gopher, the trainee, who sieved through the masses of legal papers that Mr Czul had collated for those needing copies of documented evidence for the trial. He had painstakingly filed the statements, reports, medical records and other relevant material in five-inch thick binders. He had made frantic telephone calls, booked hotel rooms and organised travelling arrangements, as well as helping Mr Czul to organise the schedule for the four-day trial. It had been a laborious and difficult task for Mr Czul and his team.

The final legal costs had amounted to an exorbitant ninety thousand pounds; an accumulation over the five years, 1993-1998, of public money and had been paid by the defendants, The Ministry of Defence. On the way to Paddington Station Mr Czul began explaining to me about 'the Distribution', how our settlement would be divided. The first recipients, The Department of Health and Social Security Compensation Recovery Unit. (CRU) would claw back thirty-five thousand pounds, money that they had paid in benefits to Chris over five years, 1990-95. She had claimed her entitlement for Invalidity Benefit, Income Support and other allowances. Then he mentioned the deduction of interim payments already made by the MOD when they first admitted liability. A further thirteen thousand pounds was allocated for Chris's parents, a payment for their role in caring for Chris during the nine months from July, 1994 to April, 1995. Then there were substantial debits to repay that we had incurred during her illness from 1989 to 1995.

The final out-of-court settlement figure amounted to four hundred and twenty thousand pounds. Rebecca and I would be left with approximately two hundred thousand pounds after all of the deductions.

TWENTY-SEVEN

Publicity

Rebecca had planned to spend four days with a school friend and was surprised when I arrived at their house to bring her home. She was obviously pleased to see me and glad that I had not had to stay in London for the duration of the trial. I explained what had happened; she was thrilled that the negligence case was finally over and that I had decided to accept the claim. But she appeared more interested in hearing about my train journey and the sights of London than my visit to the High Court.

We sat huddled together on the sofa in our home, relaxing and talking quietly. I felt weary from the day's events and mentally exhausted. I was so tired that I didn't even hear the doorbell ring. Rebecca got up to answer it and called out that there was someone asking to see me. Two men stood in the doorway. The taller one held a large camera and flash unit in his hand; the smartly dressed younger man spoke first.

"Hello, Mr Lucey. I'm sorry to trouble you, my name's Matt, and I'm from the local *Evening Advertiser*. Would you mind if I talked to you about your court case today?"

As I hadn't expected any media attention so soon, I asked him how he knew about the trial. He explained that a reporter from a news agency collected brief details on high profile court cases, which were then electronically syndicated and distributed to various tabloids nationwide. From these leads, local and national newspapers could follow up any stories that interested them. I had forgotten that my solicitor had spoken with a reporter after Judge Alliott's deliberation outside the courtroom. The interview had not lasted long and I had relinquished the opportunity to pass comment on the award, allowing Mr Czul to deal with the formalities. At the time, my mind had been preoccupied with other matters; especially the pressure imposed by the legal representatives to accept the compensation.

Now I felt mentally detached from everything around me, disorientated. It was a strange transition: a complete contrast to my feelings three hours earlier. Matt and his colleague spoke with me for only a few minutes, I think a photograph was taken but I was not paying much attention to anything that we discussed.

Next day, I arrived at the solicitor's office, an old Victorian house converted into a three-storey office building in the middle of Chippenham, Wiltshire. We continued to discuss the compensation award and Chris's will, among other business. Mr Czul specialised in personal injury claims. He was a brilliant lawyer, meticulous and informative and had always been absolutely scrupulous. He had totally condemned the stalling tactics that the opposing side used. We agreed that the litigation should have ended three years earlier when the MOD had admitted a one hundred percent liability. But there was nothing that he could have done to change the way they were allowed to drag the case all the way to the doors of the High Court.

He told me that the MOD was arranging to transfer the balance from the compensation funds to an executor's account. He would then disburse the relevant funds to those concerned. Had Christine lived, a proportion of the award would have been calculated on the basis of what she needed to adapt a home for her personal living needs, improving her quality of life. She would have been able to install various aids such as a stair lift and bath and shower accessories. Also, the funds would have enabled the provision of any necessary building conversions, as well as nursing care and domestic help. A large amount of the compensation money now represented sums to which we were entitled. It was money that we had already spent, as detailed in the Schedule of Special Damages prepared by the two separate rehabilitation agencies.

During the period between 1989 and 1995, we had accumulated

many debts, mainly through Chris's loss of earnings, £72,900, after she had had to terminate her employment in 1989. Then, in 1990 came my resignation from the dairy company, followed by twelve months off work. This represented another loss of income of £20,000. We had borrowed £15,000 to build a conservatory in which Chris could recuperate and meditate and another £10,000 to pay for our last family holiday together in Florida in 1994.

Other debts were accrued as a result of the additional cost of travelling to hospitals in Oxford, Wroughton, London and Bristol. These amounted to £5,000. Then there were my visits to Durham to see Chris and Rebecca during the nine months she stayed with her parents: thirty-five return journeys of over five hundred miles, incurring a cost of some £6,000. In addition to all this, there had been, of course, many other extra household and personal requirements. I had an annual income of £25,000 as a police constable before I resigned from full-time employment in 1997 to care for Rebecca. During the nine years between 1989 and 1998 our estimated financial loss was £153,000, a total debt of around £200,000, taking into account all of the other expenditure.

Mr Czul was interested to learn of the local media interest. I told him about another conversation I had had with the *Daily Express* newspaper group and that they were sending a reporter to my home on Thursday. I asked him if he could assist with the interview and he agreed. He was more knowledgeable than I was with the medical terminology. I did not want to get any of the details wrong.

The local newspaper reported the story that evening. The headline read: *Family Agree Compensation* and several paragraphs explained the circumstances of the out-of-court settlement. A photograph showed me holding a Mother's Day card sent to me that Rebecca had designed during a school project. The other children had teased her; they were making cards for their mums and told her she was silly because dads only got cards on Father's

Day. I suggested she should ignore them, or explain that her Dad was acting as her mother now, as well as her Father. The idea had worked. She was ten years old and capable of coping with hurtful jibes at school. I was proud that she had the courage to join in the activity: the card was a symbol of her affection for me.

The court case received media coverage and an exclusive report appeared in *The Daily Express*, on 1 April, 1998. It was my personal account of Chris's struggle to survive, the despair that resulted from the misdiagnosed smear tests and the tragic consequences. The headline read: *Agonising Testimony Of Husband Awarded A Record £420,000 Over The Error That Cost A Mother's Life.*

It went on; "as my wife lay dying she felt sorry for the doctor who missed her cancer."

The piece quoted what Chris had said in April 1993: "I was angry at the negligent events but not with the doctor who caused them. He was a nice person who had made horrendous mistakes."

It concluded with an expression of Rebecca's opinion at the time, "I feel happy that they realised what happened to Mummy wasn't fair".

This newspaper story prompted my decision to reveal and publicise the circumstances of Christine's ordeal and to warn other women of the danger of taking medical opinion too much for granted.

Rebecca and I appeared on Granada Television's *This Morning*, a popular magazine programme covering human-interest topics. We were interviewed by Richard Madelay and Julia Carling. I didn't have the chance to say everything I wanted to say referring only briefly to the misreported smear checks and the compensation award. I was pleased to get the opportunity to voice my opinion and to expose some of the details. It also gave me the chance to portray the special bond that had developed between Rebecca and myself, as a result of the fact that our lives had been in turmoil for nine years.

TWENTY-EIGHT

The clairvoyant

On 2 May, 1989, six years before she died, Chris told me she believed in life after death. It seemed a reasonable statement to make at the time. She had just returned from the operating theatre after twelve hours of gruelling surgery. Her recovery in the Intensive Care Unit was slow, her condition critical. The surgeons were very concerned that day.

Only three months earlier, she had tolerated intense hospital treatment and had suffered indescribable physical and mental pain, but this had failed to destroy her strong will to survive and her self-confidence. Chris understood her chances of survival better than most: the unpredictable physiological changes in her body and the constant fear of death led to her thinking about spiritualism and to talking to me about it. At the time I was confident of her survival because I believed she would be strong enough to overcome her ordeal. I listened tentatively as she talked about life after death.

She told me that she had realised she might die; the surgeons had discussed her operation with her and explained the many complications. Their prognosis was based on the fact that part of her tumour remained and could not be removed. This was more than enough to dishearten her and to heighten her concern about her own mortality. Chris said that if she died, she promised to watch over Rebecca and me, but first I would have to contact her spirit by saying the magic words, 'happy-go-lucky'. Then she would appear, to help and protect us.

She was convinced she would die from the trauma of her operation that day, but she found comfort in believing she could be close to Rebecca and me in the Eternal Life. She may have had a premonition. Thankfully she did not die then, she survived that ordeal and many others that followed.

I was very sceptical about spiritualism and life after death and strangely she never mentioned the subject again, until six years later. On 2 May, 1995, I stood beside Chris's hospital bed for the final time. I was cold and shaking, my body traumatised and in shock. Chris was bleeding to death and there was nothing anyone could do to save her life. I trembled uncontrollably, wiping continuous tears from my eyes, tiny droplets trickling down my face. Seeing her lying there in such a piteous state caused all the pent anxiety and stress to finally become overpowering. Six years of emotional pressure had been boiling and seething inside me. Now, here, my wife was finally facing death. There would be no reprieve this time.

At that moment I glimpsed an image of my dead father standing near to Chris. It didn't scare me, not like it had when I was ten. His body was different: it stood upright, tall and proud and flashed in front of me in mortal form, not in spirit. He smiled gently, and then he vanished. It seemed to be a message from the past, some sort of a sign to show me that Chris would be safe in the afterlife.

I composed myself momentarily and remembered Chris talking about life after death. It had been on the same day, 2 May, six years earlier. Just days before she died we had talked for a while and in a slurred, quiet voice Chris had whispered, "Don't forget… our message, Don… happy-go-lucky." She made me promise to remember it. Shortly afterwards she had become incoherent and was unable to converse sensibly with anyone else.

I considered *communicating* with Chris's spirit shortly after she died. My spiritual awareness had changed. The doubts and scepticism had disappeared: I *wanted* to believe in life after death. Psychologically I was ready to try to contact her. It was Saturday, 6 May, the day after Chris's funeral. Earlier, Rebecca had cried herself to sleep hugging Lulu, her treasured teddy bear. I concentrated for a while, my mind focusing on Chris being near me. I tried the contact message and waited for something to happen. I didn't feel embarrassed; besides no one would know, it was personal. After all, I had prayed to God when I was a child and He was invisible too. I strongly believed in Him up to the time my father died, but my faith diminished when my compulsory church attendance stopped. There was surely no difference now to those early prayers, except for the chance of seeing Chris appear in a different shape or form. There was no harm in my trying. Everyone seeks comfort at some stage in life and I was in mourning, distraught and confused.

So much had happened during Chris's illness: then that awful scene at the funeral, and the negligence case dragging on and on. My list of traumas was endless. Now I needed Chris's support in coping and coming to terms with my grief. I wanted to be strong, so that I could help Rebecca overcome her sorrow too. I was not unstable. I was in the privacy of my own home drinking tea and the house was warm now, after having been left empty and cold and for nearly two weeks. I waited patiently for something to happen, to hear her voice. But there was nothing, only silence. I abandoned any further attempt that evening.

*

Rebecca was seven years old and she had witnessed her mother's illness for six years. Nine months of that period had been spent adjusting to life in Durham. Now we were on our own, left to cope with life without Chris. It was all over, no more pain or suffering, Chris had endured enough agony and it was time to let go. I kept repeating those thoughts over and over to myself, eventually adopting a more positive attitude.

It didn't happen overnight. It took a long time, but I was determined to be strong. It was how I learnt to cope with bereavement and the dreadful memories of Chris's illness. Also, it was a philosophy that I could share with Rebecca. Chris had cheated death twice before and battled long and hard. The cancer had won in the end, but not completely. There was something it could not take.

Five years later I would experience the most startling phenomenon, which convinced me that Chris was right about her awareness of spiritual powers. On 4 April 1998, I decided to write my story about the people who were ultimately responsible for her death. Chris's determination and courage had inspired me to tell it. My crusade began in earnest, a literary journey with emotional obstacles. After eleven months I had completed my first attempt at compiling a manuscript, Then I submitted my hundred-page draft to a literary agent in London. Six months later, she informed me that it was not the right time for this particular story. I should leave it for a few years. My confidence was shattered but in October I decided to try another agent.

Their critique encouraged me and I began to rewrite my manuscript in December that year. Sixteen months later, on 12 April 2000, I was almost finished, but I was stuck. The proverbial writer's block had returned; my mind had gone blank. Up to this point I had often envisaged Chris helping me: each word was being written with some sense of her guidance. I imagined her spirit nearby, encouraging me every step of the way. Whenever I abandoned the manuscript for a few days, this thought would help me return to it with renewed zest and enthusiasm. But now I was well and truly stuck.

That evening I was looking through the script when I found myself thinking of Chris's 'happy-go-lucky' message. I had not tried these special contact words since 1995. But before I knew it, there I was asking for help again. I felt embarrassed. No extra sensory happenings had occurred in the past five years. Chris had not *appeared* to me, though I had sensed her presence. I went to bed that night thinking that I was trying to contact her like some magic genie. I had used up two of my three wishes.

The following day I found myself browsing through some complementary therapy literature in a small natural health store in a village near my home. My sister had asked me to collect some information for her. There was a clinic upstairs where therapists offered various treatments. The sweet aroma of lavender and other essential oils reminded me of the time Chris had had reflexology and massage at our home. I was deep in thought, trying to remember what my next errand was as I left the shop, when a middle-aged woman stepped out in front of me. She apologised and simply commented, "Our paths were meant to cross." I had no idea what she was talking about. I thought she was a sales assistant or a secretary. She was smartly attired and had a small, thin frame; her greying blonde hair fell to her shoulders.

Somehow we got into conversation and she explained that she was a clairvoyant. I was intrigued but did not mention anything about Chris. This woman's profession fascinated me. I had not thought about using a medium before. I had never believed in spirits or ghosts and was cautious about people who went to see clairvoyants or fortune-tellers. To my mind it was all rather like reading horoscopes: you could take it or leave it. But towards the end of Chris's life I had become interested and had learnt to respect other people's values and views on spiritual issues. I was keen to try a *reading*. I arranged to make an appointment.

The lady telephoned me at home later that morning and said she could not see me the following day but was available that afternoon. I had started writing again and did not want to be disturbed but my writing was not going terribly well. I suggested that she came to my home. We arranged an appointment for two o'clock.

The clairvoyant's name was Maureen. She told me she had practised for many years. She had discovered her skills at an early age; her mother had noticed her psychic potential when she was a child. She was well-versed in talking with the dead.

I was eager to start and sat in an armchair opposite her. She sipped water from a glass, sitting composed and then said in a soft West Country accent, "Hand me your watch, dear, or any favourite piece of jewellery you wear." I handed her my watch and looked on, waiting. She began rubbing the watch in a circular motion, first the face and then the strap. I wondered to whom she would talk if anyone. It wasn't just Chris who had died; both of my parents had passed away too. I was uneasy, not quite sure what to expect. She was quiet for a while and then said, "I'm starting to get a link. There's a lady with fair hair present. She has a pleasant soft smile… Do you know who that could be?"

"Yes," I said nervously, "it's Chris, my late wife. She passed away five years ago."

Maureen continued talking. "She wants you to know she's here. She's telling me to mention 'a rose' as proof. You will know what that means, she says."

I tried to interpret what she meant, but I couldn't remember anything about a rose.

Maureen was quiet again and in deep concentration. Seconds later, just as I was about to speak, she said, "Wait! Another spirit has joined us… another lady… this one has white hair."

"That's my Mum," I said, "she had white hair when she died, in 1997."

Since they were close when they were alive, it did not surprise me that she had turned up alongside Chris: I felt pleased and reassured that they were now together on the other side. My mood had now swung from unease to euphoria during these first few minutes of the reading. By now I was beginning to think there really *could* be something more after death. The next part of the reading would convince me further.

Maureen studied my watch; her fingers had stopped rubbing and she held it tightly. I glanced to my right, imagining two spirit silhouettes standing there together, but I was unable to define any facial or bodily features. It was like staring at two shadows but I could *feel* the presence of Christine and my Mother. I was also aware of the time: ten minutes had passed and I was eager for something more to happen.

Maureen began talking again; her voice had changed, her tone more deliberate. "Ask him about the rose that he gave me when I was in hospital, a week before I died."

I looked at Maureen again. It took a few seconds for the statement to sink in, but she didn't look at me; she carried on concentrating. I felt awkward and unsure whom I should answer. I cupped my hands over my face in disbelief as I remembered what Chris was talking about. Then I started to tell Maureen that I had taken the single rose in to Chris when she was in Dryburn Hospital, only a few days before she died. No one else had known about the flower except Chris, I explained and I had thought she was really too ill to notice.

Maureen didn't acknowledge me and waited a few minutes more before speaking again. "Dog. She mentioned something about a dog. Do you know what she means?"

I did not remember about the dog that had cheered us up by bouncing around between us, the day I told Rebecca that her Mummy had died.

"Yes," I said more confidently. "Rebecca has wanted a pet for a long time and I will get her one someday." There was silence for a while. I sat quietly with my thoughts, as though Chris were allowing me time to go through my excuses for not getting our daughter a dog.

"Well," said Maureen at last, "she's telling me she would like you to get her one."

"I will," I said, "I will." A fever of guilt washed over me. There was another long pause. Forty minutes had now gone, only twenty minutes remained of the hour-long reading.

Then Maureen said, "She's talking about a book. What does

this mean?" I told her about the manuscript I was working on, the biographical account of Chris's illness. "Well," Maureen said, "she's telling you not to worry about it; it *will* be published." She then looked towards the spot where I imagined the two spirits were standing and said, "The other lady is asking about a boy. Do you know what she's talking about?"

I tried to think about whom 'Mum' was enquiring. Maureen waited patiently for my response. I shook my head and said, "I'm sorry, I can't help, Maureen, I don't know what she means." Several more minutes of silence passed by. She sipped some water, and handed my watch back.

The session had ended. I talked to Maureen about the reading and apologised for not understanding my mother's question. She said that some spirits ask questions that are confusing and perhaps I would know the answer for the next time. Only much later did I realise that she may have been referring to me as a young boy, discovering my father's suicide.

That day with the clairvoyant I finally came face to face with the biggest mystery of life – and death. Even more strongly now, I believe Chris is watching over Rebecca and me; her spirit has survived.

That, at least, was something the cancer could not take.

POSTSCRIPT

On 14 April, 2000, I inadvertently found the help that I had needed. It would inspire me to make a final journey to the hospital were it had all begun and would assist me in bringing my story to completion. It happened after my reading with the clairvoyant.

I contacted the new proprietor of the now disused Princess Alexandra's Hospital and asked him if he would allow Rebecca and me into the deserted building. In 1996 Princess Alexandra's Hospital, formerly RAF Wroughton, had closed down and was soon to be replaced by a new Conference Centre and Housing Estate. While it was still standing, we both wanted to see the maternity ward were my daughter was born and the consultant gynaecologist's office where I was informed that her mother had cancer. My request was granted.

Before long, I found myself in the rather bizarre position of accompanying Rebecca through the deserted gynaecology ward and showing her the bed space Chris had occupied, where I had sat and cried. The room was cold and damp and the distinctive hospital antiseptic smell still lingered in the air. A lone audio remote-control unit hung absurdly on the wall behind.

We walked along the corridor to the abandoned theatres, where Chris had endured so many operations. Then we held hands as we made our way back to the main entrance. There were no tears, no outbursts of anger. We stopped and looked back along the dilapidated hospital corridor for the last time; the memories of its haunted past were entombed in its eerie silence. Soon they would be gone forever.

ENDNOTE

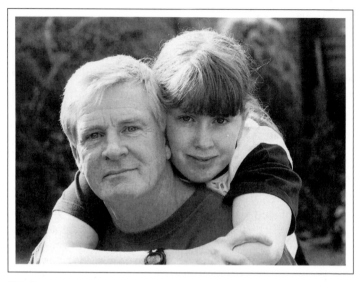

Compiling this book necessitated that I re-live the horror of its story. Now that it is finished, Rebecca and I can move on with our lives and Chris can truly rest in peace. Others can learn from her tragic ordeal. She would have wanted that. Rebecca will understand more clearly the real facts that led to the death of her mother.

Our story has been told as accurately as possible; exactly as it happened. I bear no malice or resentment. Terrible mistakes were made and those responsible will have to live with their consciences. Doctors will continue to misdiagnose their patients. When they do, they should admit they have been wrong and accept the consequences. Sometimes just a simple apology for any wrongdoing can help. That would have been a comfort to Chris; she never even blamed them for their mistakes.

Seeking to evade the truth and later admitting culpability only under duress is the ultimate insult to any victim of negligence.

Don Lucey, September 2001

APPENDICES

Chronology of Main Events in Chris's Illness

October 1982
Chris becomes ill due to a recurrence of salpingitis (inflammation of the fallopian tubes) first diagnosed in 1977.

January 1983
Endometriosis is diagnosed (the mucous membrane normally lining the womb is present in the ovaries or elsewhere). Treated with pain-killers and antibiotics.

July 1984
Chris suffers a miscarriage.

May 1986
Chris begins taking the fertility drug Clomid, resulting in a cyst and the removal of one fallopian tube.

May 1987
Chris becomes pregnant again. On examination at week 13 due to onset of bleeding, the cervix is found to be "woody".

30 January 1988
Rebecca is born. Delivery doctor recommends cone biopsy examination of abnormal cervix; overruled by gynaecologist. Postnatal bleeding does not stop and is often severe.

21 March 1988
Physical examination reveals inflamed cervix.

2 June 1988
Abnormal smear is repeated and was reported, as 'very inflammatory' Chris is increasingly concerned about the postnatal bleeding and the management of her condition.

October 1988
Chris suffers severe haemorrhage while holidaying in Portugal.

November 1988
Chris is once more assured that the postnatal bleeding is caused by hormonal imbalances due to breast-feeding or to the placenta having been stitched into the womb.

1 February 1989
Chris is admitted to hospital for a routine 'D & C' and a biopsy diagnoses invasive, terminal cancer. Chemotherapy and radiotherapy commences.

1 May 1989
Partial hysterectomy performed. Source of tumour (cervix) and lymph glands are not removed.

11 May 1989
Complications from hysterectomy: abscess is drained and faecal fistula develops in wound.

14 May 1989
Colostomy is performed. Chris now weighs five stone.

4 December 1989

Urostomy and total pelvic clearance performed, severe post-operative trauma almost resulting in death.

12 February 1990

Laparotomy and substantial abdominal repair surgery performed.

24 August 1990

Treatment under anaesthesia for substantial haemorrhaging.

8 October 1991

Gall bladder removed.

11 March 1992

Examination reveals suspected recurrence of the tumour.

Chris is told that little more can be offered in the way of treatment.

11 April 1992

A very large malignant abscess is removed during laparotomy.

Chris subsequently moves to the northeast where she continues to have treatment and management of her disability and severe pain.

2 May 1995

Chris haemorrhages to death in Dryburn Hospital.

Some aspects of cancer in general and cervical cancer in particular
by Professor Roger Cotton, Emeritus Consultant Histopathologist and Cytopathologist

There are more than two hundred different types of human cancer. Epithelial cell cancers are called carcinomas and are further categorised by the type of epithelial cell of origin and the anatomical site. Thus carcinomas of the uterus can arise in the endometrium from glandular cells and are endometrial adenocarcinomas. In the cervix adenocarcinomas also occur arising from the glandular cells lining the cervical canal.

More commonly however cervical cancers arise from squamous epithelium which covers the lowest part of the cervix and particularly the external opening of the cervix which is in continuity with the upper vagina.

It is because of this anatomical siting that sampling of the lower cervix can be satisfactorily accomplished by the taking of cervical smears with a spatula.

Natural history of cervical cancer
It has been known since the 1950's that before the potentially life-threatening symptomatic invasive carcinoma of the cervix occurs, there is a usually long period of time, often 10 - 15 years in length, when abnormalities can be found in epithelial cells removed by the use of the spatula as the "cervical smear test".

At first the differences are relatively slight, but over the years they become progressively more marked.

In this phase the abnormal cells are limited to the thickness of the epithelium and are not present in the underlying sub-epithelial connective tissues. Because the cells are confined to the epithelium this stage is know as "Pre-invasive" and present classification is cervical intra-epithelial neoplasia, new growth, shortened to CIN.

The degrees of abnormality are, somewhat artificially but very practically, divided into grades 1, 2 and 3. After a variable length of time in most cases the cells of CIN III are no longer confined to the epithelial layer and infiltrate - "invade" into adjacent tissue. Once this has happened a life-threatening situation exists due to the ability of what is now invasive carcinoma to spread deeply into tissues or to invade into lymphatic or blood vessels and spread away from the uterus to lymph nodes or other organs of the body.

If the disease is diagnosed while still pre-invasive (i.e. CIN) then with appropriate local treatment and proper follow-up the threat to life is virtually eliminated and in nearly all cases the uterus can be preserved and fertility protected.

However, if no treatment is given while only CIN is present, then treatment by surgery and/or radiotherapy is necessary and, dependent on how far the tumour has advanced (stage of tumour) length of survival is reduced. For many cancers the five-year survival figure is a useful marker.

In the case of squamous carcinoma of the cervix, illustrated five-year survival figures by stage are:

Stage 1 – confined to cervix, 85 - 95 per cent.

Stage 2 – extension directly outside cervix – 70 - 75 per cent.

Stage 3 – more severe direct extension in pelvis – 30 - 35 per cent.

Stage 4 – extension to other pelvic organs (e.g. bladder, rectum or outside pelvis) 10 per cent.

As direct spread is time- related then delay in treatment can very seriously increase mortality (death rate).

Rationale of cervical screening

The main purpose of the screening programme is to enable diagnosis and treatment of cervical abnormalities at the pre-invasive stage (CIN). Because of the long natural history of the disease (as outlined previously) testing must occur long before the invasive stage is reached and symptoms (particularly irregular uterine bleeding) has developed.

Ideally therefore testing needs to start as soon as possible after risk has occurred. Risk is very much linked to factors relevant to sexual activity, so first cervical smears should be taken soon after commencement of this landmark and repeated at regular intervals indefinitely. Infection of the cervix by certain specific strains of human papilloma virus (wart virus – HPV) which is a sexually transmitted disease is known to be a very important factor in subsequent development of the cervical cancer.

Research has identified the protective effect of differing time intervals of cervical smears and the present, and for quite a few years, recommendation of the Department of Health is for the UK Screening Programme to encourage intervals of "not more than five years" between smears. In practice many districts decide locally to offer a three-year interval. There is a considerable additional benefit from this shorter time interval.

The decision has of course to be made in the light of available resources including smear takers, trained laboratory scientists, cytopathologists and efficient computer-related administrative systems. In the United States most women have a cervical smear annually, as resources are greater but the additional benefit above a three-year programme is quite small. Of greater importance is for women to continue to avail themselves of the screening programme on a very regular basis once the risk is established.

APPENDIX C

Christine Lucey's Smear Test Results
with annotation and comment by Professor Roger Cotton, Emeritus Consultant Histopathologist and Cytopathologist

Smear Number & Date	Original Report (PMH Cytology Department)	On review in 1993	Professor Cotton's Comments
77/12865 07.11.77	Very infected smear with slight dyskaryosis. Repeat 3 months.	Mild and moderate dyskaryosis. Referral to gynaecologist for investigation.	This result was under-reported. Smear not repeated.
78/1331 08.02.78	Dyskaryotic cells throughout smear. Mild dysplasia. Repeat at six monthly intervals until it goes one way or the other.	Persistent moderate dyskaryosis – gynaecological referral now mandatory even at young age.	Second smear showing moderate dyskaryosis. Six months repeat smears very inappropriate.
81/324 06.01.81	Negative	Negative (presumed sampling problem).	There is a gap of three years between smears despite previous recommendation.
12.09.83	Sent to Bath	Not available for review	Smear discarded
1984			Smear due. No smear taken.
1985	No smear taken		
86/1223 29.1.86	Inflammatory smear. Occasional large nucleus. Repeat six months.	Some obviously atypical cells. Moderate and severe dyskaryosis. Urgent referral obligatory.	Serious under-reporting.
86/10425 18.8.86	Improved. Repeat in one year.	Technically poor with small cell yield but some moderate dyskaryosis.	Recommendation totally inappropriate.
21.03.88	Mild dyskaryoisis; atypical cells. (Patient has metaplastic postnatal background) Recommend that this be repeated at once.	Not made available for review	Urgency of repeat recognised but took 3 months
88/9245 21.06.88	Very inflammatory smear – repeat one year.	Bloodstained but frankly obvious malignant cells in clumps and singly.	Gross under-reporting. Patient was bleeding spontaneously at this time.

Explanation of terms used in previous chart

Categories of cervical smear abnormalities

BORDERLINE: Abnormalities are slight with genuine doubt about their significance relevant to the earliest stages of the disease. Agreed recommendation – repeat smear in a time span not exceeding 12 months but preferably six months.

DYSKARYOSIS: Dyskaryosis literally means abnormal nucleus. The changes in the nucleus are the most reliable indicators.

MILD DYSKARYOSIS: The changes in the cells are recognisable, relatively slight and usually involve only the more superficial layers of epithelial cells. On histology of biopsy material CIN I is usually present.

Agreed recommendations are for a repeat smear in the time span not exceeding six months though some centres would recommend investigation by colposcopy (a type of telescope which magnifies the appearances of surface cells of the cervix allowing decisions about management to be made and identifying the exact area of abnormal epithelium from which direct vision samples for histology (biopsies) can be taken).

MODERATE DYSKARYOSIS: The abnormalities are of greater degree though on biopsy the changes usually only extend as deep as two thirds of the depth of the epithelium – CIN II. Agreed recommendations are for referral for gynaecological investigation with a view to colposcopy. The patient should be seen within three months but waiting time varies according to districts and level or resources.

SEVERE DYSKARYOSIS: The abnormalities are similar to those seen in established carcinoma and the changes extend through the full thickness of the epithelium (CIN III). It is usually not possible to be sure if the cytological abnormalities are still pre-invasive or whether invasion may have already occurred and so urgent referral for investigation and colposcopy is obligatory.

It should be identified that all grades of CIN (pre-invasive carcinoma) are by themselves asymptomatic though of course women having a cervical smear taken may have gynaecological symptoms from other causes.

APPENDIX D

Useful Contacts

Bristol Cancer Help Centre
Grove House
Cornwallis Grove
Bristol
BS84PG
Information: 01179 809500
Help line: 01179 809505
Email: info@bristolcancerhelp.org
Website: www.Bristolcancerhelp.org

Wessex Cancer Trust
Bells House
11 Westwood Road
Southampton
SO17 1DL
Tel: 02380 672200
Counselling: 02380 672255
Website: www.wessexcancer.org

Macmillan Cancer Relief
Anchor House
15-19 Britten Street
London
SW3 3TZ
Tel: 020 73517811
Information: 0845 6016161
Website: http://www.macmillan.org.uk

Cancer Link
89 Albert Embankment
London,
SE1 7UQ
Tel Free line: 0808 8080000